KETO DIET

FOR WOMEN
OVER 50

The Complete Ketogenic Diet
Bible for Seniors, Living with
More Energy and Losing
Weight Quickly

NANCY TRAVIS

Table of Content

Introduction

A friend of mine recently started going through menopause. She's a few years younger than me, so I was glad to help her get through the worst of it, and to support her as she figured out these unchartered waters. The night sweats, mood swings, hot flashes, irritability, and sleep problems were all unbearable, but the weight gain was her main concern.

It's prevalent for women over 50 to gain weight as their reproductive hormones naturally decline, and their metabolism slows down (Davis et al., 2012).

Having been on the ketogenic diet for a while before I entered menopause, I thought that I wouldn't need to worry about weight gain—I've been maintaining my weight for years, and my body was fully fat-adapted (more on that later). But then I got a surprise; I, all of a sudden, got a muffin top. Only when I did some research did I find even keto would need to be adapted slightly to carry me through the transition successfully.

Another interesting facet was that I didn't experience a lot of the undesirable effects that come with menopause. Apart from a hot flash here and there, my life was continuing as normal. The fact that I was eating keto helped alleviate and prevent much of the discomfort associated with menopause.

I shared all this information with my friend, and not only did she lose the pounds she had initially gained, but she maintained her weight after following keto. And, as a bonus, her night sweats went away, and her mood stabilized.

Now it's my turn to help you. In this book, you will learn what precisely the ketogenic diet is and why staying in ketosis is essential. I'll tell you about some keto side effects which you may experience—don't worry, they don't last long—and I'll share some tried and tested tips to success.

So, without any further delay, let me show you how you can manage your waistline in your 50s.

Chapter 1: What Is the Ketogenic Diet?

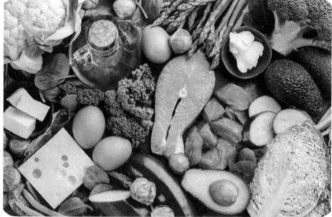

The ketogenic diet is by far one of the most popular weight-loss diets out there at the moment—and for good reason. Not only does keto help you lose and maintain your weight, but it also has tons of other benefits. These range from fighting degenerative brain diseases, improving your heart health, correcting your sleep pattern, and the list goes on (Campos, 2017).

To follow the keto diet, you'll have to limit the number of carbohydrates you eat and increase your fat and protein consumption. When you reduce your carb intake, you, in essence, take away your body's primary source of energy. This forces your body to look for fuel elsewhere, and luckily, most of us have enough fat to fuel us for quite a while. Of course, on keto, you'll also be eating more fat than usual to help maintain your energy levels.

As your body's glucose stores get depleted, your liver turns fat into ketones that then supply your body with energy. You're basically turning your body into a fat-burning machine. More than that, your body will have a constant supply of fuel, meaning you won't get tired quickly. Furthermore, eating carbs always causes your insulin to spike and with that your blood sugar to drop, which will be something of the past when you eat the keto way. By preventing this daily roller coaster of insulin, your body will function better.

How Does Ketones Work?

As I explained, glucose stores get depleted, forcing your body to look for energy elsewhere, causing your liver to break down fat into ketones, which can be used as fuel.

When your body completely relies on ketones as fuel, it means your body has switched from glucose metabolism to ketosis. The complete switchover usually takes two weeks, but it depends on how carb-heavy your diet was before you started following the keto diet. If you ate a lot of carbs beforehand, the glucose stored in your muscles will be quite full and will take longer to run out.

Although your body won't be very effective at using ketones for energy in the beginning, it will soon catch up by creating enough enzymes to convert fat into energy. It's during the time when your body is still getting used to this new way of functioning that people experience the keto flu and some lethargy. But this pass, so don't worry.

For the keto diet to be really successful, your body needs to be in ketosis all the time. This can take four weeks, four months, or longer. But as soon as you're entirely keto-adapted, you will start to see the benefits of this lifestyle. It's best to follow the keto diet for 60 days before you'll start to experience the advantages.

Once you're keto-adapted, you can increase your carb allowance to 1.76 ounces, and you won't get kicked out of ketosis. If you do have a bad day and find yourself binging on carbs, don't worry, even if your body reverts back to glucose metabolism, it will adapt to ketosis faster this time around.

Another factor to remember before you decide to increase your carb intake is the extra calories you will be consuming. If you're following the keto diet chiefly to lose weight, you'll have to keep an eye to not overshoot your daily calorie allowance.

Calories and Weight Loss

There are a lot of diets out there, but they all come down to one thing: calories in vs. calories out. To lose weight, you have to pay attention to not eating more calories than your body requires to function - any excess energy will get stored as fat.

Your body uses energy even while you're sleeping or lying around doing nothing. Your brain alone burns between 300 and 450 calories a day (Bryce, 2019).

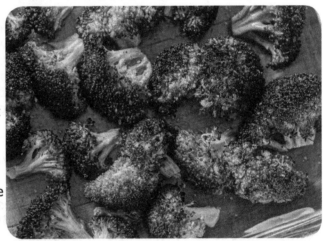

As mentioned before, carbs, fats, and proteins are made up of calories. It doesn't matter if most of your calories come from carbs, fats, or proteins; they are either used as energy or stored as fat. That means even on keto, you can overeat and gain weight. So, you will have to make sure you're eating less than what your body requires to function. There are various calorie calculators online you can use to work out your daily calorie allowance. These calculators use your age, weight, height, and daily activity level to calculate the number of calories you need to eat to lose, maintain, or gain weight.

Considering that 1 pound of fat is made up out of 3 500 calories, that means you will have to cut that amount from your diet to lose weight. Since it's generally not advised to lose more than 2 pounds a week, eating 500 calories less a day can hypothetically result in you losing 1 pound a week – barring factors like hormones, thyroid issues, and a slow metabolism hampering your progress (Calculator.net, n.d.).

Also keep in mind that not all calories are equal. If you eat 100 calories of carbohydrates, especially sugary types, it will have a different effect on your body than eating 100 calories of broccoli will have. For one, the sugar will cause a blood sugar spike and then a sudden drop, which will leave you craving more carbs. But, the broccoli won't cause a sudden increase of insulin and will keep you satiated for longer. Furthermore, the amount of broccoli you'd get for 100 calories will be significantly more than what you'd get for 100 calories' worth of carbs.

Macronutrients and Keto

Macronutrients (macros) are the fat, protein, and carbohydrates contained in the food you eat. This is where the ketogenic diet's dissimilarity to other diets is evident.

The keto diet requires you to keep your carbohydrate intake between 5% and 10% of your daily calories (Massod et al., 2020). This means you're allowed to eat anything from 0.70 to 1.7 ounces (20-50 gram) of carbs a day. Fat will make up the highest portion of your daily macros at between 55% to 60%, whereas protein will be 30% to 35%.

A sample breakdown of the macros of a 2000-calorie strict keto diet looks like:

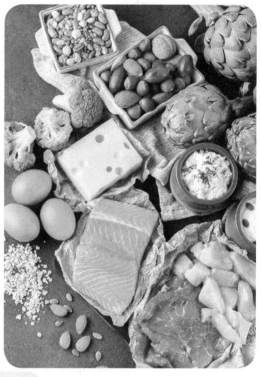

- ▨ *70% fat = 5.48 ounces (155 gram)*
- ▨ *20% protein = 4.40 ounces (124 gram)*
- ▨ *10% carbohydrates = 1.73 ounces (50 gram)*

The distinguishing factor is not so much the low carb consumption but rather a combination of low-carb with high-fat. There are diets where you eat high-protein and low-carb, but that's not what you're aiming for when you're eating the keto way. Fat plays an important role, and that is why consuming the correct balance of macros is vital.

Moreover, it will supply you with everything your body needs to run optimally.

To give you an idea of how many calories each macronutrient contains—something which is important to know if your aim is to lose weight—here's a breakdown:

- ▨ *Fat = 9 calories per 0.03 ounce (1 gram)*
- ▨ *Protein = 4 calories per 0.03 ounce (1 gram)*
- ▨ *Carbohydrate = 4 calories per 0.03 ounce (1 gram)*

Let's have a closer look at what eating fat and carbs do to your body.

Won't Eating Too Much Fat Kill Me?

The two biggest misconceptions surrounding eating fat are: It will make you fat and raise your cholesterol levels. These notions have been part of our lives for years. Remember when your mother would buy only lean meats or cut the fatty parts off? It's as if no amount of science will convince people otherwise.

Before we move to all the reasons why fat is good for you, let's first clear up the cholesterol issue.

Cholesterol has been branded as bad; the fact that it plays a crucial role in certain bodily functions is wholly ignored. People don't know that cholesterol keeps your body's cells in good condition, and it produces certain hormones, vitamin D, and bile that plays a role in digesting fat. In fact, all cells create cholesterol, and only a moderate amount of the cholesterol in your blood comes from the food you eat. As you can see, lowering your cholesterol is not everything it is chalked up to be, and it may even damage your body (Zampelas & Magriplis, 2019).

Let's look at the different types of cholesterol to get a better idea of what we should avoid.

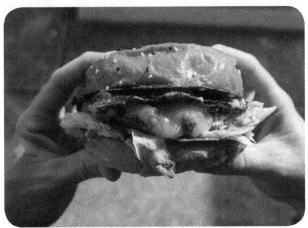

High-density lipoproteins (HDL) are the good guys, while low-density lipoproteins (LDL) are the dangerous type. However, not everyone knows that LDL comes in two sizes A and B. Pattern A is the large, fluffy (non-dangerous) type, and pattern B is small and dense and tends to cling to the walls of your arteries, causing damage. When we're told to eat plant-based processed oils instead of animal fats because it will reduce the bad cholesterol, they don't tell you that it's the good part of the bad cholesterol that gets broken down and the dangerous pattern B that ends up increasing.

When you have a low LDL count, there's less 'traffic' in your bloodstream, meaning having pattern B particles won't be that harmful. But, as soon as your LDL count rises, the chances of oxidation increase, and the bad particles will stick to your arteries and cause damage. On the other hand, where pattern A may be larger particles, they're softer, meaning everything can move freely in your bloodstream, and there's no chance of oxidation.

Research has actually proven that a diet high in animal fat is healthier and more effective than a low-fat diet (Manikam, 2008).

Fat is essential, not only because it provides your body with energy, but it also performs a number of other vital functions, including:

▨ Helps absorb fat-soluble vitamins A, D, E, and K
▨ Controls inflammation
▨ Maintains health of cells

Another benefit of eating enough fat is the fact that it keeps you satiated for longer. This is important if you're trying to lose weight and beat any cravings.

Fat is absorbed in the body and, after being digested, is broken down into fatty acids and glycerol. Saturated and unsaturated long-chain fatty acids are packed with cholesterol and proteins and get stored as fat. Short-chain and medium-chain fatty acids, on the other hand, go directly to the liver where they're used as a quick energy source in the form of ketones.

It's clear that not all fats are equal.

Why is Overeating Carbohydrates Bad?

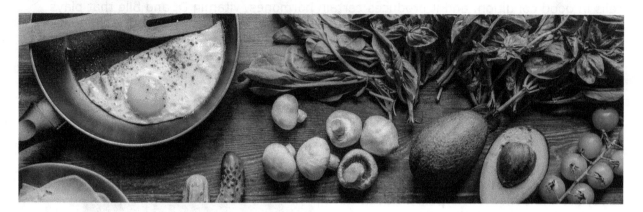

There are heaps of studies into carbohydrates, but not a lot of them cover the ideal amount to eat. Add to that the fact that the available information can be somewhat contradictory and hence, confusing, it's difficult to know what's up and what's down.

Then there's the issue of processed carbohydrates and those that occur naturally in fruits, vegetables, grains, milk, etc.

On the ketogenic diet you will eat some carbs; it is actually impossible to cut out all carbs unless you go to the extreme and follow the carnivore diet. The main carbs you're warned against on the keto diet are simple carbs, chiefly that of a processed nature.

So, what happens when we eat carbs? Firstly, carbohydrates are converted into glucose, which is the main source of fuel if you have glucose metabolism. If you're keto, that's the opposite of what you want. You want your body to run on your fat stores, a metabolic state called ketosis.

If you eat too many carbs, your glucose stores will never get depleted, and you won't be able to go into ketosis. But that's not the only negative thing about overeating carbs.

Carbs are delicious, but you pay dearly for such comfort food in the form of calories. Although calories aren't fundamentally bad since your body needs calories to function, it can lead to weight gain. And when you're over 50, you want to pay extra attention to your calorie intake to keep the pounds from piling on.

What about the effect of carbohydrates on your blood sugar?

Carbs and Your Blood Sugar

Most carbs digest quickly. This leads to a sudden rise of your blood sugar levels. In an effort to lower your blood sugar, your body releases insulin, but instead of releasing just enough, it overcompensates, which leads to an almost instant drop in blood sugar levels. When this happens, you feel lethargic, and believe it or not, hungry.

This blood sugar roller coaster will, over time, affect your body's ability to control its blood sugar levels. This increases your risk of developing insulin resistance and, consequently, type 2 diabetes (Dyson, 2015).

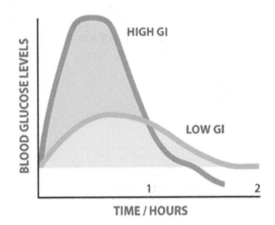

Blood sugar levels also increase your risk of heart disease. This constant spike and drop enhance the possibility of bad cholesterols particles becoming oxidized and subsequently damaging your blood vessels (Jackson, 2017).

Two main factors impact the exact amount of carbs to eat: your goals and your body's composition. Let's say you have type 2 diabetes; then I suggest you eat as few carbs as you can to get your blood glucose and insulin resistance to improve faster. If you're trying to lose weight, the more you restrict your carb intake, the quicker you will lose weight. But, I'm sure that you'll agree that's easier said than done. When it comes to restrictive diets, failure is almost guaranteed – unless you have an extra dose of willpower. So, maybe increase your carbs if you feel like you're going to fall off the wagon, but make sure it stays below 1,7 ounces; otherwise, it's not keto anymore but actually just low carb.

It's worth mentioning that it will be harder for your body to go into ketosis, the more carbohydrates you eat.

Okay, I've mentioned ketones and ketosis a lot, and you may be interested in what ketones are and how ketosis works. I think it's time to break it down for you.

Chapter 2: Eating the Keto Way

When building the perfect meal plan you have to remember that keto is low-carb, not no-carb. In the previous chapter, we covered the macros, and it is vital to your success that you stay within those percentages. If you neglect either your fat or protein intake, you won't get all the necessary nutrients to make your body efficiently heal itself and that includes losing weight.

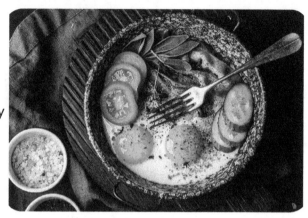

Foods to Eat

Meat	The meat on your plate should be unprocessed. That is the only way you'll know you're not eating any hidden carbs. Smoked meat, sausages, cold cuts, and other processed types of meat oftentimes contain more carbohydrates than you're allowed to eat. Check the label. If the carb percentage is below five, then you can eat it. I suggest you avoid it altogether because these types of meat usually have a lot of preservatives, which isn't good for your health either. Go for organic, grass-fed meat if you can.
Fish and Seafood	Since fat plays such an integral part in the keto diet, choose fatty fish. Salmon, tuna, herring, mackerel, and sardines are great choices. Fish covered in a crust is a no-no as the carb content will be too high.
Eggs	You're allowed to eat eggs daily in whichever way you fancy. Eggs are a great source of protein and contain not even close to an ounce of carbs. I especially like scrambling my eggs in butter and adding a tablespoon or two cream. Delicious!
Vegetables	Don't be fooled into thinking that the keto diet is made up of copious amounts of meat—especially bacon—eggs, cheese, without any vegetables. I know that is what you see on social media, but it's not correct. Vegetables play a very important role in the keto diet. Not only do they fill you up, but they're also a great source of fiber, something you'll need, particularly if you're over 50. The only veggies you're not allowed to eat are root vegetables. Veggies that grow under the ground, such as carrots, beetroot, potatoes, and sweet potatoes, contain a lot of carbs. Opt for greens (usually containing fewer carbs) such as spinach, kale, broccoli, and zucchini. Cauliflower will also be a staple in your house since it is so versatile you can even turn it into a crispy pizza base.

Fruit	Unfortunately, you'll have to limit yourself to eating fruits. Most fruits contain a lot of sugar and are high in carbs, whereas berries have less than 5% carbohydrates. I like eating my berries with some cream. It is the perfect way to get rid of any sugar cravings. Berries are nature's candy.
Oil	Fat is your friend when you're on the keto diet. You will consume fat from meat, eggs, avocado, etc. but don't forget the oil you cook your food in. Coconut oil, avocado oil, olive oil will make an appearance in recipes over and over again. You'll also use a lot of butter in your cooking.
Full-fat Dairy	Full-fat is the key here. Also, use cream instead of milk. Although there's less than an ounce of carbs in a glass of milk, it quickly adds up. Flavored yogurt also contains a lot of hidden sugars and carbs and doesn't have a lot of probiotics, so the full-fat unsweetened kind is preferred.
Nuts	Nuts are allowed, but considering that they're high in calories, moderation is key. It's no use if you're following a keto diet, but snacking on nuts is ruining your progress. Cashews are particularly high in not only calories but carbs. Macadamia, Brazil, and pecan nuts are ideal choices.

Here is a breakdown of food that will help you reach your carb, fat, and protein quote for the day.

Carbohydrates (5-10% of your calories)	Protein (10-20% of your daily calories)	Fat (70-80% of your calories)
Based on a 2 000-calorie diet, you're looking at 0.9 -1.76 ounces (25-50 grams).	Based on a 2 000-calorie diet, you're allowed to eat 1.8 -3.5 ounces (50-100 grams).	Based on a 2 000-calorie diet, you should eat 5.5-6.3 ounces (150-170 grams).
⬥ Eggplant ⬥ Asparagus ⬥ Tomatoes ⬥ Broccoli ⬥ Spinach ⬥ Cauliflower ⬥ Cucumber ⬥ Kale ⬥ Zucchini ⬥ Green beans ⬥ Bell peppers ⬥ Brussel sprouts ⬥ Celery	⬥ Chicken ⬥ Turkey ⬥ Beef ⬥ Lamb ⬥ Venison ⬥ Pork ⬥ Salmon ⬥ Sardines ⬥ Tune ⬥ Shrimp ⬥ Eggs	⬥ Avocado oil ⬥ Olive oil ⬥ Flaxseeds ⬥ Olives ⬥ Avocados ⬥ Pumpkin seeds ⬥ Sesame seeds ⬥ Hemp seeds ⬥ Nuts ⬥ Nut butters (natural, no added sugar ⬥ Coconut ⬥ Cheese (not processed) ⬥ Ricotta cheese ⬥ Cottage cheese ⬥ Plain full-fat yogurt ⬥ Cream

Drinks on the Menu

Lucky for the coffee and tea lovers among you, you're allowed to drink as many of these beverages as you want—without sugar and milk, of course. Milk contains a lot of carbs, so if you can't stand black coffee or tea, a splash of cream is more than okay. Then there's the big kahuna of drinks—bulletproof coffee. This mix of coffee, butter, and oil will give you an energy kick of note while keeping hunger at bay. A lot of people drink this instead of eating breakfast. I do caution against overindulging; you will gain weight. Also, considering that you're drinking your calories, you may not even realize when you've overshot your calorie count for the day and won't have any left to spend on real food.

Bone broth is another favorite of mine, mainly to replenish some of the salt and electrolytes you will lose on the keto diet. It also contains a lot of nutrients, which are good for you.

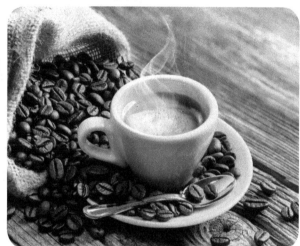

Then, not surprisingly, water is by far the best thing when it comes to quenching your thirst. It contains zero calories, so you can drink as much as you want. Add some lemon or cucumber slices, mint, or anything else you think will add some flavor to water.

When it comes to alcohol, a glass of wine will do no harm, but beer is out. Spirits like tequila, whiskey, and vodka are carb-free, but that doesn't give you free rein to go wild. These drinks do contain calories, so keep that in mind before you get ready for a big night out with friends.

Before we go on to the "bad bin" of foods, I have to take a moment to discuss artificial sweeteners. On the ketogenic diet you're allowed to sweeten your coffee or tea with sugar substitutes. But, just because it's permitted doesn't mean you should do it. These sweeteners come with adverse effects; they can cause cravings, trigger insulin release, and when you eat, you may not be able to taste the natural sweetness of food.

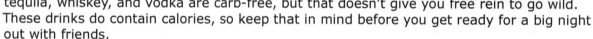

Foods Not to Eat

On the keto diet, the two main things that are forbidden are, you guessed it, sugar and carbs. Of course, there are thousands of foods on the market that fall under those two categories, which makes things somewhat confusing. Then we have the subsets of both, with some being worse than others.

Sugar

Sugar has never really been considered healthy. Research time and time again has shown that not only does sugar contribute to obesity; it even increases the mortality rate due to cardiovascular disease (Howard & Wylie-Rosett, 2002).

Fructose was for a long time considered healthy, but in actual fact it may be worse than glucose. Where glucose is converted into glycogen and stored for later use, fructose cannot be used as energy. The liver consequently converts it into fat (triglycerides). The excess triglycerides trigger insulin resistance, which can later lead to type 2 diabetes—not to mention the numerous other adverse effects it has on your body.

Understandably this makes sugar a big no-no on the ketogenic diet. Soft drinks, fruit juice, flavored water, and sports drinks should be avoided. The same applies to chocolate, candy, cakes, cookies, and all-American favorite, breakfast cereal. If you're not sure how much sugar a product contains, just check the label; if you see it listed in the top three ingredients, you can be sure that the product is loaded with sugar. Even still, there are a lot of hidden sugar alcohols in foods, so I suggest avoiding anything that comes in a package and looks sweet.

Fruit also falls in this category—it is full of sugar and high in carbs and shouldn't be part of your diet.

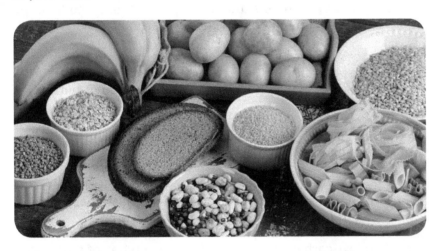

Carbohydrates

Carbs can be divided into three classes: sugars, starches, and fiber. In turn, these are separated into simple or complex carbs.

Simple carbs are broken down quickly by the body to be used as energy.

Complex carbs are made up of sugar molecules that are strung together in long, complex chains. Complex carbohydrates are found in foods such as peas, beans, whole grains, and vegetables.

When it comes to choosing between the two, natural should always win. You will have to keep in mind that you're following a keto diet, and that means even though natural, single-ingredient carbs are okay in general, they're not okay for you. For example, root vegetables, whole grains, and most fruit fall under good carbs, but they're not allowed if you're eating low carb.

Good carbs	Bad carbs
◈ Vegetables (including those that grow underground) ◈ Fruit ◈ Legumes ◈ Nuts ◈ Whole grain ◈ Seeds	◈ Sugary drinks ◈ White bread ◈ Cookies, cakes, and pastries ◈ Ice cream ◈ Chocolate ◈ Fruit juice ◈ Candy ◈ French fries and potato chips

When calculating your carbohydrate intake, you should always think of "net" or digestible carbs. This means the fiber content is not counted toward your overall carb consumption. This means you will be able to eat more actual carbs. Also, there's no limit on the amount of fiber in your diet, so eat your fill of low-carb veggies (Lattimer & Haub, 2010).

However, net carbs on labels of processed foods are a whole different story. This usually just means the product contains hidden sugar alcohols – blood sugar spikes guaranteed. It's best to avoid processed foods altogether; that way you know exactly what you're putting into your body.

That was a long way of saying bread, pasta, oats, potatoes, rice, muesli, whole grain, and other starches (good or bad) aren't allowed on the keto diet.

I do want to end off with a warning. The ketogenic diet is popular, and as with most 'trendy' things, companies are quick to think of ways to milk the system. This means store shelves are packed with 'keto-friendly' and low-carb products. But on closer inspection of the label, you will find that these foods aren't what they claim to be. So, don't fall in their trap. Avoid packaged foods even when low-carb claims are made. These types of foods are counter-intuitive to your weight loss in any case. Natural is always the preferred option.

Chapter 3: Keto for Women Over 50

In this chapter, you will find out why women who are over 50 will have to make some adjustments to the ketogenic diet. Since a woman's body goes through a lot of changes during that time, a different approach is needed. But don't worry, it's not that big a shift. I will also cover how you can slow down the aging process by eating less, but more nutritious food.

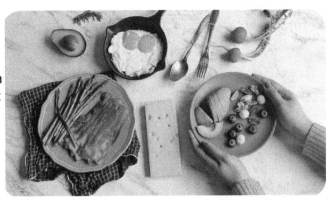

What Keto Does to a Woman's Body

We've already established that the ketogenic diet has various positive health benefits. But are there any advantages specific for women over 50? Although most of the research done on keto is based on the effects on men, a respectable number focused chiefly on women. The results indicate that keto is definitely a worthwhile diet for older women.

Helps Control Blood Glucose

Stable blood sugar levels are important. Excess insulin throws out essential hormones that regulate ovulation. Considering that insulin resistance, obesity, and type 2 diabetes often go hand in hand, getting your blood glucose levels under control and losing weight will get you one step closer to conceiving.

As we know, keto doesn't cause the blood sugar spikes, which leads to weight gain and type 2 diabetes. In fact, studies done explicitly on women found that over four months, obese women with type 2 diabetes not only lost a lot of weight, but their fasting blood sugar and hemoglobin A1c (HbA1c) also improved markedly (Goday et al., 2016). The HbA1c count is a good indication of long-term blood glucose control.

Helps with Depression

A 2019 study found that the keto diet, in combination with psychotherapy and regular exercise, cured a 65-year-old woman's depression. She had had type 2 diabetes and clinical depression for 26 years, but as soon as she started eating low carb and her Hba1c dropped, she no longer had type 2 diabetes, and her depression was gone (Cox et al., 2019).

Reduces Inflammation in the Body

Inflammation is very dangerous; it harms cells in the body. Cardiovascular disease is only one of the many adverse effects of inflammation.

Less severe consequences include skin outbreaks, weight gain, lethargy, and body aches. A lot of women experience these daily because the carbohydrate consumption that is part of the standard American diet triggers inflammatory pathways. Since you won't be eating carbs on keto, inflammation is stopped in its tracks.

Relieves Symptoms of Menopause

As menopause draws near, estrogen levels drop. When this happens, women get hot flashes, battle depression, experience mood swings, and gain weight. But, when you eat keto, you will be consuming foods that increase estrogen, including broccoli and cauliflower, sesame seeds, flaxseeds, and walnuts.

Complements Cancer Treatment

Research has found that a ketogenic diet is beneficial to cancer patients (Branco et al., 2016). A study of 45 women who were diagnosed with endometrial or ovarian cancer found that keto decreased insulin-like growth factor (IGF-I) in the body. This hormone is claimed to encourage the spread of cancer (Cohen et al., 2018). Scientists believe the decrease of IGF-I and blood glucose creates an unreceptive environment for cancer cells.

Effective in Treating PCOS

Polycystic ovarian syndrome affects as many as 5 million American women of reproductive age. Still, the negative impact on health continues well into menopause and beyond (Centers for Disease Control and Prevention, n.d.). Since eating keto promotes weight loss—one of the primary factors in managing PCOS—hormone levels will return to normal, and for women who are still of child-bearing age, falling pregnant becomes more likely (McGrice & Porter, 2017).

Even though there are numerous health benefits to following the ketogenic diet, it may not be healthy for everyone.

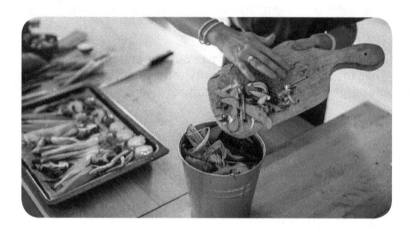

Women who suffer from the following should not attempt to eat low carb without the guidance of a health professional:

◈ Liver of kidney failure
◈ Alcohol or drug abuse
◈ Type 1 diabetes
◈ Pancreatitis
◈ Disorders that affect fat metabolism
◈ Carnitine deficiency

✳ **Additionally, women who are pregnant or breastfeeding should avoid eating keto.**

The Gender and Age Difference

I mentioned earlier how not a lot of keto studies have been done on female subjects. There's still a lot we don't know. Yes, it is possible to reason that lower blood sugar levels and subsequent insulin regulation can prevent diabetes, but it still amounts to guesswork. That being said, the limited studies that have been done found there are significant differences between the two genders and how they react to keto. The main factor that contributes to these dissimilarities comes down to hormones.

Hormones and Keto

As a woman, you know that if your hormones are out of balance, then your life is too. Hormones are a fundamental part of every process in a woman's body, from reproduction to stress management. It doesn't help that they tend to fluctuate during various times of the month, and due to other reasons, such as a lack of sleep.

Although men have hormones too, they're not nearly as sensitive to change. And keto is a pretty drastic change, so women have to pay extra attention to how they feel.

When you first switch over to eating low carb, the following may occur:

You may experience a lower sex drive, vaginal dryness, moodiness, and insomnia. This is due to low estrogen levels caused by cutting out processed foods containing soybean oil, which promote estrogen production, or due to menopause. If you want to raise your estrogen levels—which I recommend doing when you're over 50—eat more fat.

Keto may also increase the stress hormone cortisol. When your body realizes it doesn't have enough glucose in its system, it triggers a stress response and cortisol is released. This chronic stress may lead to an imbalance of blood glucose levels, decreased bone density, and a loss of muscle. But, considering that eating carbohydrates also causes fluctuating blood sugar levels, and a slew of other things, extra cortisol is not the worst that could happen.

The Menstrual Cycle

This is another thing women have to face, and men don't. I know you may be thinking why include the menstrual cycle if this book is targeted at women 50 years and older. Well, late-onset menopause is a reality. Some women may continue to menstruate even after the age of 55 (AsiaOne, n.d.).

What makes periods extra difficult when you're following keto is the powerful cravings, which makes eating low carb particularly challenging.

Other than that, you feel bloated, and you're holding on to more water than usual—this reflects on the scale which is in itself, discouraging. You get headaches, which may turn into a keto headache if you don't pay attention to your electrolyte balance and stay hydrated.

Digestion is an issue, and you more than likely feel like eating a bowl of pasta instead of meat and veggies packed with fiber. And then there are the cramps…

This is why so many women fall off the keto bandwagon at that time of the month—something men won't understand.

What Your Body Needs After 50

If you're 50, you're most likely in menopause or very close to it. As your hormone levels shift, your body changes. You won't be able to stop this process, but if you respond to these changes correctly, you may be able to slow it down!

Here are some changes you can expect when you hit the 50 year mark, and how you can use keto to give your body what it needs to stay healthy.

Your metabolism will slow down: A slower metabolism means it will take fewer calories for you to gain weight. The high-fat aspect of keto curbs any hunger pangs, and you will automatically eat less to counter a sluggish metabolism.

Hormonal changes may cause digestive issues: Cutting carbohydrates from your diet will promote a healthy gut, which will ease issues like irritable bowel disease or other inflammatory bowel issues.

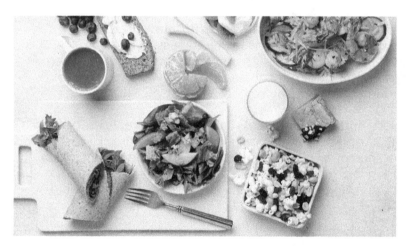

Bone loss accelerates: The drop in estrogen as you approach or enter menopause is to blame for a loss of bone density. Exercise will help, but eating foods that raise your estrogen levels is also a good idea. The ketogenic diet contains a lot of these foods, among them kale and olives.

Your body stores more fat: Fat, protein, and enough fiber will kill any cravings you have and will make it easier to avoid temptation. If you don't eat in excess, there won't be fat for your body to hold on to.

Your skin changes: Bone broth is a great source of collagen, which helps your skin maintain its elasticity.

Your libido declines: Removing sugary foods and carbs from your diet will help boost your sex drive.

Calcium deficiency becomes a reality: The ketogenic diet allows you to eat dairy, but furthermore, kale, and broccoli, which are staple low-carb veggies, are high in calcium.

A lot of what we experience as we grow older isn't pleasant, but it is in our power to not only make it more bearable but to slow the whole process down.

It's already evident that following a wholesome, nutritious diet will prolong your life by eliminating and preventing dangerous diseases. But calorie restriction also has the ability not only to increase your life but your lifespan. Here's how.

In one study, participants were asked to eat 15% fewer calories for two years. After the time elapsed, researchers found that not only were their metabolisms slower (meaning their bodies were more energy efficient), they also had less oxidative stress (Redman et al., 2018).

Cutting calories can even reduce your risk of getting age-related diseases.

It all comes down to slowing your basal metabolism. According to Redman and associates, if a person's metabolism is slow, energy is spent more economically, which means cells and organs can 'work' less, and this increases their longevity. Although there are other factors, such as oxidative stress and dietary and biological elements that influence your metabolism, cutting calories is an excellent way to get it where healthy aging is possible.

Keto Challenges After 50

It's no wonder that your body will react adversely when you first start keto; cutting carbs from your diet basically turns everything upside down. It all of a sudden has to learn to use ketones as fuel instead of glucose. So, during this transition, you may not feel your greatest. Almost everyone who starts keto experiences some or all of these symptoms:

- Nausea
- Fatigue
- Headache
- Keto flu
- Irritability
- Lack of motivation
- Sugar cravings
- Brain fog
- Dizziness
- Keto rash
- Constipation
- Diarrhea

But, since you're a woman over 50, you may have to face some extra stumbling blocks, chiefly:

Your weight loss plateaus: If this happens, up your fat consumption to the 80% mark.

Hormone imbalances: Don't restrict your calories too much and don't lose too much weight. A woman's body is healthiest with 22 to 29 percent body fat. Another way to combat these pesky hormones is to sync your diet with your menstrual cycle. When your period starts, eat more protein, then from days 6 to 11, go to the extreme end of low carb, and on days 12 to 16 eat a lot of avocado, broccoli, garlic and parsley. You can end your cycle (days 17 to 28) by eating moderate low carb.

How to Maintain Ketosis

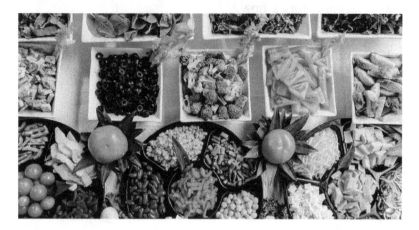

In short—don't cheat. You will see that a lot of people recommend you take a day off and have a cheat meal. If you're serious about eating low-carb, you'll resist the urge to do this. The main reason is that it increases the chance of your body reverting back to glucose metabolism, which means you will have to suffer to get back into ketosis again. Granted, it may take less time the second or third time around, but do you really want to put your body through that much stress?

Armed with all the knowledge of the adverse effects carbohydrates and sugar have on your body, cheating shouldn't be an option. The fact of the matter is, keto is not a diet; it is a lifestyle change.

That being said, you still live in the real world where you have to go to social gatherings and special events where food will inevitably be involved. These situations should not be used as an excuse to eat what you want without keeping your macros in mind. If that is your approach, you can kiss ketosis goodbye for a while and prepare yourself for another keto flu as your body battles its way through carb overload.

To stay true to your diet, no matter what the situation, do two things.
1. Track your carb intake
2. Test your ketone levels

If you do this, you will be 100% sure you're not going over your carb allowance for the day and that you're actually still on track.

Other than that, using what you know about the keto diet to guide you, i.e., no processed sugar or starchy food, then you should be able to stay in ketosis permanently.

If you have, however, overindulged and consequently gave your body access to an easy fuel source—glucose—there are ways you can get back into ketosis faster.

◈ Eat only 5% carbs
◈ Get active
◈ Increase your fat intake (MCT oil is a good source)
◈ Try intermittent fasting
◈ Exercise on an empty stomach

Chapter 4: Getting Started the Keto Diet

We've covered all the nitty-gritty details of the ketogenic diet for women over 50. Now it is time to get down to business—getting you started on keto. There are a few tips and tricks that I found made my transition a stress-free one. This includes ditching all the non-keto food and restocking my kitchen with low-carb staples. I have some rules to share with you that will guarantee your success.

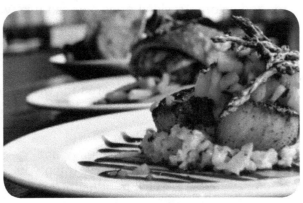

7 Rules to Success

1. Preplan Your Diet

If you're prepared, you'll eliminate the chance of you throwing your hands up in the air and giving up before you drive to the nearest fast-food restaurant. If you pre-plan what you're going to eat throughout the week, it will also make shopping a much more straightforward process. You'll have a shopping list to work from and won't aimlessly wander through the aisles.

2. Prep Your Meals

If you're a busy woman and don't have time to spend hours a day in the kitchen, or maybe you just don't like cooking that much, meal prep may be the answer to your problems. When I first started eating keto, I found it convenient if I cooked a week's worth of meals every Sunday. It's an excellent way to make sure you don't use the excuse "I don't have time to cook" as a reason to eat processed and carb-heavy foods.

3. Take it Slow

Getting into ketosis and staying there is not going to happen overnight. Persistence will win over extreme carb-cutting that will lead you crashing and burning a few days into the keto diet. Similarly, don't expect to see the positive health benefits immediately and then feel discouraged if you don't. You can't expect to undo a lifetime's worth of damage in only a few days.

4. Try Intermittent Fasting

If you do want to speed the process up in a healthy manner, you can try intermittent fasting. This will get you into ketosis faster, meaning all the healing processes will start sooner than expected. The premise of intermittent fasting is you'll only have a window of X number of hours to eat in, and the rest of the time nothing that contains any calories is allowed. There are different timeframes, for example, 16/8, which means you'll fast for 16 hours and eat for 8.

5. Ignore the Scale

Women have this weird love affair with bathroom scales—they just can't leave them alone. Want to know a secret? They're actually pretty useless considering that your weight fluctuates throughout the month, depending on where in your cycle you are and how much water you're holding back. Various other factors also influence the number on the scale. Let's say you've decided to weight train. Well, the day after training when your muscles are sore, you'll weigh more!

6. Keep a Food Journal

This isn't even a recommendation but an instruction, especially in the beginning. There is no way you'll know how many carbs you're eating if you don't make a note of them. Now, when I say journal, I don't mean you have to write everything down on paper. There are carb and calorie tracking apps you can use, which will do all the hard work for you. I mean, calculating net carbs, protein, and fat sounds like a complicated and tedious task.

Another reason why I think food journals are terrific is that it gives you an idea of what time during the day you experience cravings, or when you're hungriest. If you have that information, you can be prepared for when it happens and have a healthy snack on hand.

7. Clean Out Your Kitchen

Getting rid of all the carb-heavy and sugary foods is probably the best thing you can do for yourself. You'll be maximizing your chances for success since you won't have easy access to unhealthy foods.

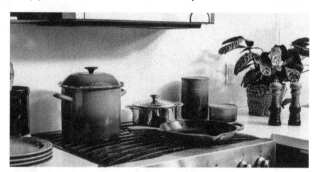

Here's a list of foods that you should get rid of and then ban from your house!

Fridge and Freezer	Pantry
◈ Fruit juice	◈ Chocolate
◈ Soda	◈ Muffins
◈ Margarine	◈ Breakfast cereals
◈ Store-bought salsas	◈ Sugar of any kind
◈ Any low-fat items	◈ Cookies
◈ Jam	◈ Potato chips
◈ Cakes	◈ 'Healthy' processed snacks (granola bars, etc.)
◈ Store-bought waffles	◈ Dried fruit
◈ Buns	◈ Crackers
◈ Ice creams	◈ Popcorn
◈ Ketchup	◈ Candy
◈ Ready-made spice mixes	◈ Wheat flour
	◈ Bagels
	◈ Rice
	◈ Bread
	◈ Pasta
	◈ Canned soup
	◈ Beans

This list isn't extensive—that would take pages and pages—but it includes some of the most popular high carb and sugary foods in American households. I suggest you read the labels on any remaining food you're not sure of. If it contains any sugar or carbs, ditch it.

Keto Staples

Okay, I'm not going to leave you with an empty kitchen. Here's a list of items you can restock your kitchen with.

Quick protein sources	Cooking essentials
◈ Beef jerky	◈ Coconut flour
◈ Salami	◈ Almond flour
◈ Pepperoni	◈ Sesame flour
◈ Canned fish (tuna, salmon, sardines)	◈ Shredded coconut
◈ Smoked oysters	◈ Cacao butter
◈ Cheese	◈ Ground flaxseed
◈ Eggs	◈ Chia seeds
◈ Pork rinds	◈ Pink Himalayan sea salt
◈ Healthy keto fats	◈ Baking soda
◈ Extra virgin olive oil	◈ Baking powder
◈ Ghee	◈ Cream of tartar
◈ Avocado oil	◈ Gelatin
◈ Coconut oil	◈ Bone broth
◈ Butter	◈ Xanthan gum
	◈ Extracts (apple, vanilla, maple, lemon, caramel, etc.)
	◈ Stevia
	◈ Monk Fruit sweetener
	◈ Sugar-free dark chocolate chips
	◈ 85% dark chocolate
	◈ Whey protein powder

Vegetables and Fruit	Condiments
◈ Asparagus	◈ Low-carb (and sugar-free) salad dressing
◈ Brussels sprouts	◈ Sugar-free ketchup
◈ Cauliflower	◈ Hollandaise sauce
◈ Celery	
◈ Cucumber	
◈ Green beans	
◈ Broccoli	**Snacks**
◈ Spinach	
◈ Olives	
◈ Cabbage	◈ Macadamia nuts
◈ Blueberries	◈ Pecans
◈ Kale	◈ Almonds
◈ Peppers (red and green)	◈ Walnuts
◈ Swiss chard	◈ Unsweetened peanut butter
◈ Zucchini	◈ Unsweetened almond butter
◈ Avocado (technically a fruit)	◈ Unsweetened coconut butter
◈ Lettuce	◈ Seeds (pumpkin and sunflower)
◈ Tomatoes	◈ Olives

Prepare Your Kitchen

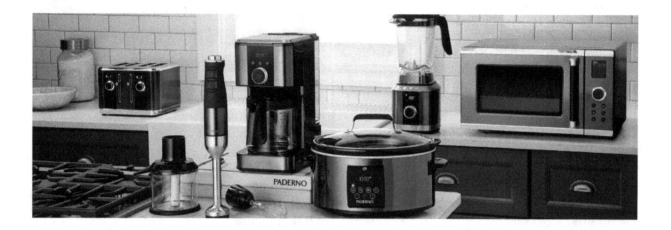

Before I move on to the recipes, I want to list some of my most-used gadgets to cook keto-friendly meals. I'm by no means suggesting that you have to have all of this in your kitchen to follow the ketogenic diet successfully, so please don't go out and buy anything you won't use.

You'll see I'm not listing cutlery and crockery and other items commonly found in a kitchen. I think in your 50 years on earth, you've spent enough time in a kitchen to know the basics required to cook food.

Kitchen scales: Out of all the things on the list, this is one I would highly recommend buying. In the beginning, you won't be able to eyeball your macros as the more experienced keto dieters can. You will have to use a kitchen scale to weigh your food to know how much you are eating. You can then punch these numbers into a carb and calorie tracker app, and it will let you know if you're on track.

Storage and food prep containers: Essential for meal prepping and storing leftovers.

Slow cooker: If you plan on prepping your meals in advance, I suggest investing in a slow cooker. You're able to cook a large amount of food at once and then divide it into portions for the week. If meal prepping is not your thing, you can still use the slow cooker to prepare a keto-friendly meal in a fraction of the time.

Spiralizers: This is a nifty little gadget if you want to fool your eyes into thinking you're eating pasta. You can spiral different veggies into forms and sizes that resemble spaghetti, fettuccine, or other shapes.

Egg cooker: Okay, you'll soon come to find that you'll be eating more eggs than usual. They're high in fat and protein and low in carbs, and that makes eggs a great snack. Boil a few eggs, pop them in the fridge and enjoy when you're feeling a little peckish.

Immersion blender: This is a baby food processor that you can hold in your hands to blitz up smoothies, make your own Hollandaise sauce, ground nuts, or whip some cream to add to your coffee. Just make sure you buy one with multiple attachments.

Frying pan/skillet: You'll be eating a lot of steaks, so why not get a frying pan or skillet to cook it in?

Roasting pan: A whole chicken or beef roast surrounded by veggies, roasted in the oven, and then covered in a creamy cheese sauce. Doesn't sound like you're on a diet, does it? A roasting pan is a perfect container to make delicious meals in the oven.

Safety First

As this chapter ends and you get ready to try out some of my top keto recipes, just a reminder to put your safety first. It's possible to get so wrapped up in what you're doing that you forget some standard safety rules. This is dangerous when you're working with open flames, boiling water, steam, and knives.

I think a lot of people don't know how to handle knives safely because they try to mimic cutting techniques they see on TV. I remember I once showed off my non-existent chopping skills and almost lost a finger.

So allow me to run you through a quick crash course in knife safety.

◈ Always use a cutting board. Don't cut anything while holding it in your hand.
◈ Do not leave knives lying around in the sink. Clean them as soon as possible and put them away.
◈ Don't store knives loose in a drawer. You may be reaching for something else and then get a nasty surprise.
◈ Dull knives cause more injuries. Always use a sharp knife.
◈ On the hand that's holding the item that is being cut, curl your fingers under. If you keep them straight, they'll be in the way.
◈ Always point the knife away from you; blade facing down. Don't run or fool around with a knife in your hand.
◈ Keep your focus while you're chopping, dicing, or mincing.
◈ If you drop a knife, don't try to catch it. Step back and let it fall.

Okay, for you to look through the recipes, find one you like, and head to the kitchen! I hope you found the information in this book helpful and feel that you now know enough to start the ketogenic diet confidently. I promise you—speaking as a woman over 50—this diet will change your life for the better.

Chocolate American Pancakes

Macros: Fat 92% | Protein 4% | Carbs 4%
Prep time: 15 minutes | Cook time: 12 minutes | Serves: 4

Really, you can treat yourself to breakfast, as you will for a dessert. These pieces are straightforward to make, yet delightful and soothing for a morning chill. You can top the pancakes with some raspberries for better tastes.

2 cups (250 g) almond flour
2 tsp baking powder
2 tbsp erythritol
¾ tsp salt

2 eggs
1 1/3 cups (320 ml) almond milk
2 tbsp butter + more for frying

Topping:
2 tbsp unsweetened chocolate buttons
Sugar-free maple syrup

4 tbsp semi-salted butter

1. In a medium bowl, mix the almond flour, baking powder, erythritol, and salt.
2. Whisk the eggs, almond milk, and butter in another bowl. Add the mixture to the dry ingredients and combine until smooth.
3. Melt about 1 ½ tablespoons of butter in a non-stick skillet, pour in portions of the batter to make small circles, about 2 pieces per batch (approximately ¼ cup of batter each). Sprinkle some chocolate buttons on top and cook for 1 to 2 minutes or until set beneath. Turn the pancakes and cook for 1 more minute or until set.
4. Remove the pancakes onto a plate and make more with the remaining ingredients. Work with more butter and reduce the heat as needed to prevent sticking and burning.
5. Drizzle the pancakes with some maple syrup, top with more butter (as desired) and enjoy!

TIPS:
Storage: Put excess pancakes in a Tupperware and refrigerate for up to a week.
Reheat: Warm in the microwave for 30 to 60 seconds.
Serve it with: Top with some fresh raspberries for improved tastes and enjoy with warm almond milk or coffee.

NUTRITIONAL FACTS PER SERVING:
Calories: 1065 | Total Fat: 111.67g | Carbs: 10.4g | Fiber: 5.9g | Protein 12.95g

Pancetta Sandwiches with Lemony Frisée

Macros: Fat 81% | Protein 17% | Carbs 2%
Prep time: 15 minutes | Cook time: 21 minutes | Serves: 4

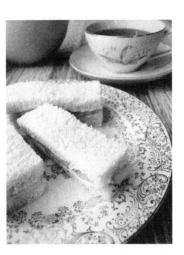

A catchy sandwich shouldn't be a duty. This set is one that is ready in little time, fresh, crunchy, and packed with lots of flavor for a morning boost. Frisée with vinegar may not sound like a regular for the morning, but give this sandwich a shot and start testifying of the goodness.

8 pancetta slices
4 eggs
1 tbsp water
Salt and black pepper to taste
4 Monterey Jack cheese slices

4 oz (100 g) frisée lettuce
1 tsp vinegar
4 low-carb English muffins, split
Olive oil for frying and drizzling

1. Preheat the oven to 425°F/220°C and line a baking tray with greaseproof paper.
2. Lay the pancetta slices on top without overlapping and bake for 8 to 12 minutes, turning halfway until golden brown and crispy. Take out of the oven and drain the pancetta pieces on a paper towel-line plate.
3. In a bowl, whisk the eggs with the water, salt, and black pepper. Heat 1 teaspoon of olive oil in a non-stick skillet over medium heat and pour in a quarter of the egg mix. Cook for 45 seconds or until set beneath. Turn the egg and lay a cheese slice in the center. Fold the edges of the eggs over the cheese (about 1 to 1 ½-inches in). Cook for about 1 minute or until the cheese melts. Remove the egg onto a plate and set aside. Repeat the process for the remaining eggs and cheese slices.
4. In a bowl, toss the frisée lettuce with the vinegar, salt, and about 2 teaspoons of olive oil.
5. Toast the muffins in a clean non-stick skillet for 1 minute or until golden brown and start assembling the sandwiches.
6. Divide the frisée lettuce on the bottom parts of the muffins, lay an egg set on each, then two pancetta slices each, and cover with the top parts of the muffins. Serve immediately.

TIPS:
Storage: Preserve remaining sandwich in a Tupperware and refrigerate for up to a day.
Reheat: Take out the lettuce. Separately warm bread, pancetta, and egg in microwave. About 30 to 45 seconds per batch. After, re-assemble the sandwich and enjoy.
Serve it with: Enjoy the sandwiches with a glass of coffee or fresh berry juice.

NUTRITIONAL FACTS PER SERVING:
Calories: 475 | Total Fat: 43.47g | Carbs: 2.4g | Fiber: 0.3g | Protein 19.32g

Turmeric Nut Loaf with Zesty Cream Cheese

Macros: Fat 85% | Protein 10% | Carbs 5%
Prep time: 25 minutes | Cook time: 45 minutes | Serves: 6

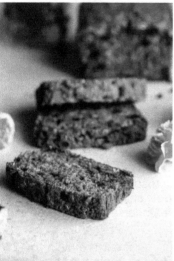

A rightly-flavored bread that bursts with sunshine energy. It is dense with compact but moist crumbs to make a slice or two fill you well. The cream cheese topping is everything! You may even add some cinnamon powder to the topping to kick up the aroma.

4 eggs, separated
1 cup (160 g) swerve sugar, divided
1 stick (100 g) butter, room temperature
½ tsp salt, divided
½ cup (113.5g) almond flour
½ cup (113.5g) ground almonds

1 tsp turmeric powder + extra for garnish
A pinch cinnamon powder
1 tsp baking powder
1 tsp fresh lemon zest
1 tbsp plain vinegar
3 tbsp sugar-free maple syrup
7 oz (200 g) cream cheese

1. Preheat the oven to 350°F/175°C and line a loaf pan with grease-proof paper. Set aside.
2. Using electric beaters, whisk the egg whites and half of the swerve sugar until stiff.
3. Add the remaining swerve sugar, butter, salt, and whisk until smooth.
4. Pour in the egg yolks, almond flour, ground almonds, turmeric powder, cinnamon powder, baking powder, lemon zest, and two-thirds of the vinegar. Mix until smooth batter forms.
5. Pour the batter into the loaf pan and level the top with a spatula. Bake for 45 minutes or until a small skewer inserted comes out with moist crumbs and not wet batter.
6. Remove the pan and allow the bread cool in the pan.
7. Meanwhile, in a medium bowl, mix the maple syrup, cream cheese, and remaining vinegar until smooth.
8. Remove the bread onto a cutting board and spread the topping on top. Garnish with the lemon zest and pistachios. Slice and serve.

TIPS:
Storage: Put bread in a plastic loaf container and refrigerate for up to 1 week.
Reheat: No re-heating needed.
Serve it with: Enjoy with omelet, tea, coffee, or fresh berry juice

NUTRITIONAL FACTS PER SERVING:
Calories: 573 | Total Fat: 55.96g | Carbs: 7.68g | Fiber: 3g | Protein 13.74g

Green Shakshuka

Macros: Fat 78% | Protein 17% | Carbs 5%
Prep time: 15 minutes | Cook time: 9 minutes | Serves: 4

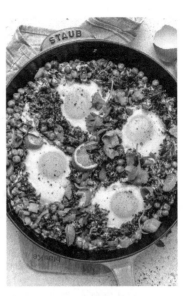

My Russian friend made this version of her shakshuka and I asked for the recipe immediately. It doesn't only taste amazing from the infusion of minty herbs, but it is completely keto-certified. It makes you so salivated that you can't stop digging in.

1 tbsp olive oil
2 tbsp almond oil
½ medium green bell pepper, deseeded and chopped
1 celery stalk, chopped
¼ cup (57 g) green beans, chopped
1 garlic clove, minced

2 tbsp fresh mint leaves
3 tbsp fresh parsley leaves
½ cup (113 g) baby kale
¼ tsp plain vinegar
Salt and black pepper to taste
¼ tsp nutmeg powder
7 oz (200 g) feta cheese, divided
4 eggs

1. Heat the olive oil and almond oil in a medium frying pan over medium heat.
2. Add the bell pepper, celery, green beans, and sauté for 5 minutes or until the vegetables soften.
3. Stir in the garlic, mint leaves, 2 tablespoons of parsley, and cook until fragrant, 1 minute.
4. Add the kale, vinegar, and mix. Once the kale starts wilting, season with salt, black pepper, nutmeg powder, and stir in half of the feta cheese. Cook for 1 to 2 minutes.
5. After, use the spatula to create four holes in the food and crack an egg into each hole. Cook until the egg whites set but the yolks still running. Season the eggs with salt and black pepper.
6. Turn the heat off and scatter the remaining feta cheese on top. Garnish with the remaining parsley and serve the shakshuka immediately.

TIPS:
Storage: Keep remaining shakshuka in a Tupperware and preserve in the fridge for up to 2 days.
Reheat: Warm food (covered) in the microwave for 30 to 60 seconds.
Serve it with: Serve with low-carb toasts.

NUTRITIONAL FACTS PER SERVING:
Calories: 322 | Total Fat: 28.42g | Carbs: 4.1g | Fiber: 0.6g | Protein 13.01g

Fruity Breakfast in a Jar

Macros: Fat 92% | Protein 3% | Carbs 5%
Prep time: 10 minutes | Cook time: 0 minute | Serves: 4

Sometimes a quick breakfast fix is the right way to start the morning. These jars are straightforward to assemble and taste excellent. They can be pre-made the night before, so they are ready to enjoy right out of bed.

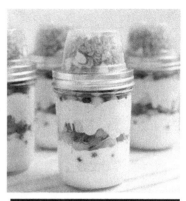

3 cups (681 g) Greek yogurt, room temperature or chilled
8 tbsp sugar-free maple syrup
½ cup (113 g) mixed seeds
½ cup (113 g) mixed berries, frozen or fresh
4 medium jars

1. Start by sectioning the ingredients into half. We will be making two layers of the ingredients.
2. Divide half cup of the Greek yogurt between the four jars.
3. Then, share half of the remaining ingredients on top: maple syrup, mixed seeds, and berries.
4. Repeat the layer a second time with the rest of the ingredients.
5. Dig spoons in and enjoy!

NUTRITIONAL FACTS PER SERVING:
Calories: 334 | Total Fat: 34.83g | Carbs: 4.57g | Fiber: 1.5g | Protein 2.59g

TIPS:
Storage: This meal finishes up in one sitting, they are that good! However, to store, cover the jars with a tight lid and refrigerate for up to two days.
Reheat: None needed.
Serve it with: For more textures, enjoy the jars with some almond flour pancakes.

Herby Goat Cheese Frittata

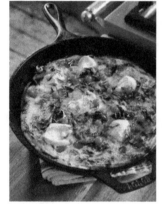

Macros: Fat 78% | Protein 18% | Carbs 4%
Prep time: 15 minutes | Cook time: 15 minutes | Serves: 4

Move dinner all the way down to breakfast and have a feast. A loaded frittata is a sure way to boost your energy ahead for the day's activity. This rich piece of egg is also an excellent post workout meal.

1 tbsp avocado oil for frying
2 oz (56 g) bacon slices, chopped
1 medium red bell pepper, deseeded and chopped
1 small yellow onion, chopped
2 scallions, chopped
1 tbsp chopped fresh chives
Salt and black pepper to taste
8 eggs, beaten
1 tbsp unsweetened almond milk
1 tbsp chopped fresh parsley
3 ½ oz (100 g) goat cheese, divided
¾ oz (20 g) grated Parmesan cheese

TIPS:
Storage: Keep excess frittata in a Tupperware and refrigerate for up to 3 days for maintained freshness.
Reheat: Warm frittata in the microwave.
Serve it with: It serves better with tomato-arugula salad.

1. Preheat the oven to 350°F/175°C.
2. Heat the avocado oil in a medium cast-iron pan and cook the bacon for 5 minutes or until golden brown. Stir in the bell pepper, onion, scallions, and chives. Cook for 3 to 4 minutes or until the vegetables soften. Season with salt and black pepper.
3. In a bowl, beat the eggs with the almond milk and parsley. Pour the mixture over the vegetables, stirring to spread out well. Share half of the goat cheese on top.
4. Once the eggs start to set, divide the remaining goat cheese on top, season with salt, black pepper, and place the pan in the oven. Bake for 5 to 6 minutes or until the eggs set all around.
5. Take out the pan, scatter the Parmesan cheese on top, slice and serve warm.

NUTRITIONAL FACTS PER SERVING:
Calories: 494| Total Fat: 43.27g| Carbs: 5.09g| Fiber: 0.9g| Protein 20.67g

Breakfast Toast in a Bowl

Macros: Fat 80% | Protein 18% | Carbs 2%
Prep time: 15 minutes | Cook time: 30 minutes | Serves: 4

A breakfast platter is more deserving than two pieces of toast and a splatter of butter. And when you're not up for a spread, bake the different foods in a bowl and enjoy as a whole.

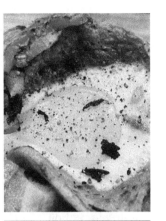

4 tbsp butter + greasing
1 tbsp chopped fresh basil
12 salami slices
8 tomato slices

4 low-carb bread slices
4 eggs
Salt and black pepper to taste

1. Preheat the oven to 300°F/150°C.
2. Heat 1 tablespoon of butter in a skillet over medium heat and sauté the basil until fragrant. Stir in the salami and cook for 3 minutes per side or until golden brown. Remove the salami and basil to a plate and set aside.
3. Put the tomatoes in the pan and cook for 3 to 5 minutes per side or until brown around the edges.
4. Brush 4 medium ramekins with some butter and press a bread slice into each bowl to line the walls of the ramekins. If the bread tears in the middle, that's okay.
5. Place one salami each in the center of each bread and then two salamis each against the walls of the ramekin that doesn't have complete bread covering. The goal is to create a cup of food in the ramekins either with bread or salami.
6. Divide the tomatoes into the bread cup and crack an egg into the center of the food cup. Bake in the oven until the egg whites set but the yolks still running.
7. Take out the ramekins, season with salt, black pepper, and serve immediately.

TIPS:
Storage: Keep remaining food in the ramekin and cover with foil. Refrigerate for up to a day.
Reheat: Warm food covered in the microwave or preheated oven.
Serve it with: Have a good wash down with tea, warm almond milk, or coffee.

NUTRITIONAL FACTS PER SERVING:
Calories: 290 | Total Fat: 25.85g | Carbs: 1.41g Fiber: 0.2g | Protein 12.57g

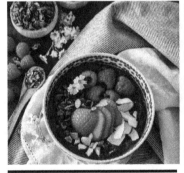

TIPS:
Storage: Place remaining food in a bowl with an airtight lid and cover. Refrigerate for up to 3 days.
Reheat: No reheating required.
Serve it with: Add some seeds and more berries for a better medley.

Cocoa and Berry Breakfast Bowl

Macros: Fat 95% | Protein 1% | Carbs 4%
Prep time: 10 minutes | Cook time: 0 minutes | Serves: 2

Quick fixes are the way to true enjoyment! There's nothing better than tossing a few chilled ingredients into a bowl and digging in immediately. Cocoa, berries, and nuts are a pretty family and taste well together.

½ cup (113.5 g) strawberries, fresh or frozen
½ cup (113.5 g) blueberries, fresh or frozen
1 cup (240 ml) unsweetened

almond milk
Sugar-free maple syrup to taste
2 tbsp unsweetened cocoa powder
1 tbsp cashew nuts for topping

1. Divide the berries into 4 serving bowls and pour on the almond milk.
2. Drizzle with the maple syrup and sprinkle the cocoa powder on top, a tablespoon per bowl.
3. Top with the cashew nuts and enjoy immediately.

NUTRITIONAL FACTS PER SERVING:
Calories: 520 | Total Fat: 56.02g | Carbs: 7.15g | Fiber: 2.2g | Protein 1.06g

Poached Avocado Toasts

Macros: Fat 83% | Protein 12% | Carbs 5%
Prep time: 15 minutes | Cook time: 5 minutes |
Serves: 4

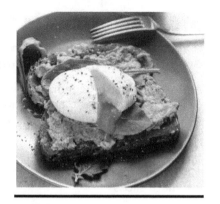

Here is an opportunity to make your toasts more exciting. Avocados bring on a good worth of healthy fats to the dish; an addition that serves as a creamy blend between bread pieces and gorgeous poached eggs.

4 eggs
4 slices low-carb bread
½ avocado, pitted and peeled
1 tbsp almond oil
1 tbsp cream cheese, room

temperature
1 tbsp heavy cream
Salt and black pepper to taste
1 cup (160 g) baby spinach

1. Bring about 3 cups of water to a rolling boil, crack in an egg, and poach for 30 seconds to 1 minute. Use a slotted spoon to remove the egg onto a paper towel-lined plate and set aside. Poach the remaining three eggs the same way.
2. Place the bread slices in a toaster and let brown for about 1 minute.
3. Meanwhile, mash the avocado in a bowl and mix with the almond oil, cream cheese, heavy cream, salt and black pepper.
4. When the bread is ready, spread some avocado on one side of each bread slice, stick some spinach on top, and spread the remaining avocado on the leaves. Add an egg each, season with salt, black pepper, and enjoy immediately.

NUTRITIONAL FACTS PER SERVING:
Calories: 237 | Total Fat: 22.28g | Carbs: 3.31g | Fiber: 1.8g
Protein 6.94g

TIPS:
Storage: Separate eggs, spinach, mashed avocado, and bread into separate bowls. Cover and refrigerate for up to 1 day.
Reheat: Warm the bread in a preheated oven for 5 to 10 minutes. For the eggs, boil some water and turn the heat off. Place the egg in the water to reheat for 30 to 60 seconds. After re-assemble the toast and enjoy.
Serve it with: Add some cheddar cheese to the toast and serve with fresh berry juice for added tastes.

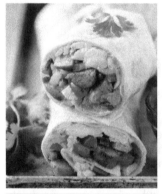

Eggs and Cheddar Breakfast Burritos

Macros: Fat 71% | Protein 24% | Carbs 4%
Prep time: 15 minutes | Cook time: 6 minutes | Serves: 4

An easy way to work burritos into your morning routine and still maintain a light balance. Swap the meats for some eggs and vegetables, enhance with some white cheddar cheese, and enjoy!

3 tbsp butter
2 small yellow onions, chopped
½ medium orange bell pepper, deseeded and chopped
10 eggs, beaten
Salt and black pepper to taste

8 tbsp grated cheddar cheese (white and sharp)
4 (8-inch) low-carb soft tortillas
2 tbsp chopped fresh scallions
Hot sauce for serving

TIPS:
Storage: Wrap excess burritos in foil and refrigerate for up to 3 days.
Reheat: Warm burritos in the microwave.
Serve it with:
Serve with julienned vegetables like sweet bell peppers and celery.

1. Melt the butter in a skillet over medium heat and stir-fry the onions and bell pepper for 3 minutes or until softened.
2. Pour the eggs into the pan, let set for 15 seconds and then, scramble. Season with salt, black pepper, and stir in the cheddar cheese. Cook until the cheese melts.
3. Lay out the tortillas, divide the eggs on top, and sprinkle some scallions and hot sauce on top. Fold two edges of each tortilla in and tightly roll the other ends over the filling. Slice into halves and enjoy the burritos.

NUTRITIONAL FACTS PER SERVING:
Calories: 478 | Total Fat: 38.09g | Carbs: 5.56g | Fiber: 0.8g | Protein 27.92g

Cheese Fondue with Low-Carb Croutons

Macros: Fat 75% | Protein 24% | Carbs 1%
Prep time: 15 minutes | Cook time: 15 minutes | Serves: 4

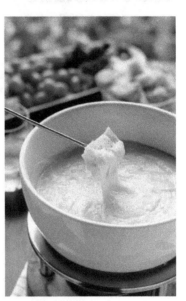

My granny taught me to go hard on a treat when I get the opportunity to splurge. Cheese fondue is my way of diving deep into the ocean of cheeses and pampering myself dirty. Luckily, we need all the fatty elements that the blend of cheeses offer; therefore, it is a win-win for us!

1 garlic clove, halved
1 cup (227 g) dry white wine
14 oz (400 g) grated Mexican cheese blend
10 oz (283 g) grated Monterey Jack cheese
10 oz (283 g) grated cheddar cheese (white and sharp)

1 tbsp fresh vinegar
¼ tsp nutmeg powder
Black pepper to taste
1 tbsp xanthan gum mixed with 2 drops of water
3 tbsp butter
1 low-carb bread loaf, cut into 1-inch cubes

1. Rub the inner part of a pot with the garlic and pour in the white wine. Cook over low heat until warm.
2. Slowly add the cheeses while gently stirring in one direction until the cheeses melt.
3. Stir in the vinegar, nutmeg powder, and black pepper.
4. If the mixture is too thin, add the xanthan gum and stir in the same direction until thickened. Pour the cheese fondue into a serving bowl and set aside for serving.
5. Melt the butter in a skillet and toast the bread cubes on both sides until golden brown and slightly crunchy.
6. Serve the cheese fondue with the low-carb bread pieces.

TIPS:
Storage: Keep leftovers covered in a bowl and chilled in the fridge for up to 5 days.
Reheat: Warm both cheese fondue and low-carb bread cubes in a preheated oven before re-serving.
Serve it with: Enjoy the cheese fondue with celery and sweet peppers sticks as options.

NUTRITIONAL FACTS PER SERVING:
Calories: 1147 | Total Fat: 95.54g | Carbs: 4.02g | Fiber: 0g | Protein 68.11g

Avocado Deviled Eggs with Mayo Sauce and Prosciutto

Macros: Fat 83% | Protein 13% | Carbs 4%
Prep time: 20 minutes | Cook time: 8 minutes | Serves: 4

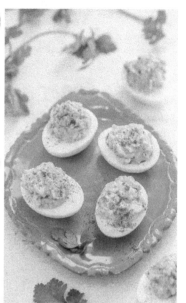

Deviled eggs remain a classic for pre-servings. Interestingly, the egg white holes allow for an endless option of filling. Avocado infused yolks add a good twist. Meanwhile, check out the flare of excluding mayonnaise in the filling, but creating a dipping sauce to compliment the eggs.

4 eggs
Ice bath
4 prosciutto slices, chopped
1 avocado, pitted and peeled
1 tbsp mustard
1 tsp plain vinegar
1 tbsp heavy cream

1 tbsp chopped fresh cilantro
Salt and black pepper to taste
½ cup (113 g) mayonnaise
1 tbsp coconut cream
¼ tsp cayenne pepper
1 tbsp avocado oil
1 tbsp chopped fresh parsley

1. Boil the eggs in a pot of water over medium heat for 7 to 8 minutes. Remove the eggs into the ice bath, let sit for 3 minutes and then peel the eggs. Slice the eggs lengthwise into halves and empty the egg yolks into a bowl. Arrange the egg whites on a plate with the hole side facing upwards.
2. While the eggs cooked, heat a non-stick skillet over medium heat and cook the prosciutto on for 5 to 8 minutes or until golden brown and crispy. Remove the prosciutto onto a paper towel-lined plate to drain grease.
3. Add the avocado to the egg yolks and mash both ingredients with a fork until smooth. Mix in the mustard, vinegar, heavy cream, cilantro, salt, and black pepper until well-blended. Spoon the mixture into a piping bag and press the mixture into the egg holes until well-filled.
4. In a bowl, whisk the mayonnaise, coconut cream, cayenne pepper, and avocado oil.
5. On serving plates, spoon some of the mayonnaise sauce and slightly smear out the sauce in circular movement. Top with the deviled eggs, scatter the prosciutto on top and garnish with the parsley. Enjoy immediately.

TIPS:
Storage: Chill deviled eggs and sauces separately in bowls and chill for up to a day.
Reheat: None required.
Serve it with: For more fatty elements, top the deviled eggs with grated Parmesan cheese and enjoy.

NUTRITIONAL FACTS PER SERVING:
Calories: 381 | Total Fat: 35.59g | Carbs: 3.71g | Fiber: 2g | Protein 12.47g

Blue Cheese and Peperonata Crostini

Macros: Fat 82% | Protein 16% | Carbs 3%
Prep time: 20 minutes | Cook time: 15 minutes | Serves: 4

Crostini has forcefully taken on the identity of wine-flavored tomato topping. Make a change and improve your crostini serving. Blue cheese is the right guy for the facelift as whisked with heavy cream to increase the fatty element of the meal.

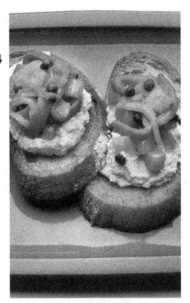

4 low-carb bread slices, cut into halves lengthwise
1 tbsp olive oil + extra for brushing
3 tbsp melted butter
½ medium red bell pepper, deseeded and sliced
½ small yellow onion, sliced
1 garlic clove, crushed
½ (7 oz) (198 g) can crushed tomatoes

¼ tsp dried thyme
¼ tsp dried rosemary
Salt and black pepper to taste
1 tbsp almond milk
1 lemon, zested
1 tsp plain vinegar
2 cups crumbled blue cheese
2 tbsp heavy cream
1 tbsp chopped fresh basil to garnish

1. Preheat the oven to 300°F/150°C and line a baking tray with greaseproof paper.
2. Arrange the bread pieces on the baking tray, brush with some olive oil, butter, and toast in the oven for 8 to 10 minutes or until golden brown.
3. Meanwhile, heat the olive oil in a pot and sauté the bell pepper, onion, and garlic for 5 minutes or until the vegetables are tender. Stir in the tomatoes and season with the thyme, rosemary, salt, and black pepper. Cover and cook for 10 minutes or until the tomatoes become tender.
4. Turn the heat off and add the almond milk, lemon zest, vinegar, and use an immersion blender to puree the ingredients until smooth. Set aside.
5. In a bowl, mix the blue cheese and heavy cream.
6. Take the bread out of the oven, arrange on a serving platter, and brush with some more olive oil. Spread the blue cheese mix on each bread and top with the peperonata (bell pepper sauce). Garnish with the basil and enjoy.

TIPS:
Storage: Keep bread and sauces separately preserved in bowls in the refrigerator for up to 4 days.
Reheat: Warm the bread and peperonata in the microwave before assembling to serve.
Serve it with: Top the crostini with some chopped avocados for increased healthy fats.

NUTRITIONAL FACTS PER SERVING:
Calories: 406 | Total Fat: 37.66g | Carbs: 2.91g | Fiber: 0.5g | Protein 14.95g

Cheese Patties with Raspberry Dip

Macros: Fat 86% | Protein 12% | Carbs 2%
Prep time: 15 minutes | Cook time: 4 minutes | Serves: 4

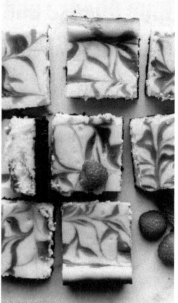

I love cheesecakes so much and try not to share when I drag myself to making one. However, I found a way to make cheesecake at ease and incorporate them into my snacking routine too. This altered way to make a cheesecake follows a pancake-making pattern and pairs it with a tasty raspberry dip. Enjoy!

Cheesecakes:

1 2/3 cups (400 g) goat cheese
1/3 cup (68 g) grated Monterey Jack cheese
2 egg yolks
¼ cup (50 g) swerve sugar

½ cup (100 g) almond flour
2 tbsp (30 g) xanthan gum
1 tsp (10 g) vanilla extract
3 tbsp olive oil for frying

Raspberry dip:

1 cup (200 g) fresh raspberries
2 tbsp swerve sugar

Mint leaves for garnish

Cheesecakes:

1. In a bowl, mix the goat cheese, Monterey Jack cheese, egg yolks, swerve sugar, almond flour, xanthan gum, and vanilla until well-combined. Shape the mixture into a dough and divide into 6 to 8 (2-inch thick) patties.
2. Heat the olive oil in a non-stick skillet over low heat, and fry the cheese patties on both sides for 1 to 2 minutes per side or until golden brown and compacted.
3. Remove the cheesecakes to a paper towel-lined plate to drain grease and set aside.

Raspberry dip:

1. In a food processor, add the raspberries, swerve sugar, and blend until smooth.
2. Pour the mixture into a serving bowl, garnish with the mint leaves and enjoy with the cheesecakes.

TIPS:

Storage: Keep leftover cheesecakes in a bowl (covered) and refrigerate for up to 2 days. Store raspberry dip in the fridge too.
Reheat: Slightly warm cheesecake in the microwave before enjoying again.
Serve it with: Swap raspberries for strawberries or blueberries for a change. You can also use feta and Gruyere cheeses for the cakes.

NUTRITIONAL FACTS PER SERVING:
Calories: 615 | Total Fat: 59.72g | Carbs: 2.72g | Fiber: 1g | Protein 17.69g

Cheesy Guacamole with Veggie Sticks

Macros: Fat 79% | Protein 16% | Carbs 4%
Prep time: 10 minutes | Cook time: 0 minutes | Serves: 4

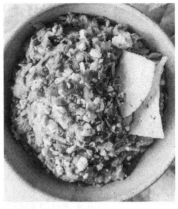

Guacamole reminds of cheering moments when friends gather and share good times. I attended a Mexican group study ones and loved the spicy effects that the guacamole there had. So, I tried it at home, improved it with some cheddar cheese, cumin powder and was proud of myself. Here's the recipe for you!

12 avocados, peeled and pitted
½ small tomato, diced
1 tbsp chopped fresh cilantro
1 green chili, deseeded and minced
1 tsp cumin powder
1 ½ cups grated cheddar cheese

3 tbsp butter
1 tsp vinegar
Salt and black pepper to taste
2 celery stick, cut into thirds
1 small sweet red bell pepper, deseeded and julienned

1. Mash the avocado in a bowl using a fork or masher until smooth.
2. Mix in the tomatoes, cilantro, green chili, cumin powder, cheddar cheese, butter, vinegar, salt, and black pepper.
3. Serve the guacamole with the celery sticks and bell pepper strips. Enjoy!

TIPS:
Storage: Refrigerate leftover guacamole and veggies for up to 4 days.
Reheat: None required
Serve it with: Spread guacamole on low-carb toasts for a flare.

NUTRITIONAL FACTS PER SERVING:
Calories: 307 | Total Fat: 27.32g | Carbs: 3.56g | Fiber: 1.5g | Protein 12.59g

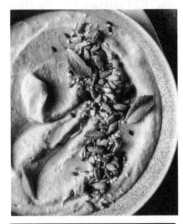

TIPS:
Storage: Preserve leftovers covered in a bowl and chill in the fridge for up to a week.
Reheat: None required.
Serve it with: Enjoy the hummus with celery sticks or low-carb tortilla chips.

Minty Hummus

Macros: Fat 88% | Protein 8% | Carbs 4%
Prep time: 15 minutes | Cook time: 15 minutes | Serves: 4

A hummus blend that reminds us of the romance of the Mediterranean area. It is a simple combination, which includes avocado for that fat-lifting effect.

½ (132.5 g) cauliflower, cut into florets
1 tbsp almond oil
Salt to taste
¼ avocado, chopped
¼ cup (57 g) fresh mint leaves + extra for garnish
¼ cup (57 g) fresh parsley leaves
½ tbsp plain vinegar

1 garlic clove, crushed
1 tbsp pure tahini
1 cup heavy cream
½ cup grated Monterey Jack cheese
2 tbsp butter
½ tsp cumin powder
2 tsp water or enough for thinning

1. Preheat the oven to 350°F/175°C and line a baking tray with foil.
2. Place the cauliflower on top, drizzle the almond oil on top and season with salt. Use your hands to rub the seasoning well on the cauliflower. Roast in the oven for 10 to 15 minutes or until the cauliflower is golden brown and tender.
3. Remove the cauliflower from the oven into a food processor and top with the avocado, mint leaves, parsley, vinegar, garlic, tahini, heavy cream, Monterey Jack cheese, butter, cumin powder, and water. Blend until smooth and adjust the taste with salt.
4. Pour the hummus onto a serving plate and garnish with some mint leaves.

NUTRITIONAL FACTS PER SERVING:
Calories: 291 | Total Fat: 29.16g | Carbs: 3.35g | Fiber: 1.3g | Protein 5.82g

Tempura Zucchinis with Cream Cheese Dip

Macros: Fat 91% | Protein 5% | Carbs 4%
Prep time: 5 minutes | Cook time: 10 minutes | Serves: 4

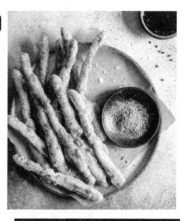

Swap shrimps for tempura and watch your guests "wow" at you for the creativity. They taste as good except that these zucchini option introduces more greens into your pre-main serves. That's a good thing, isn't it?

Tempura zucchinis:
1 ½ cups (200 g) almond flour
2 tbsp heavy cream
1 tsp salt
2 tbsp olive oil + extra for frying

1 ¼ cups (300 ml) water
½ tbsp sugar-free maple syrup
2 large zucchinis, cut into 1-inch thick strips

Cream cheese dip:
8 oz cream cheese, room temperature
½ cup (113 g) sour cream

1 tsp taco seasoning
1 scallion, chopped
1 green chili, deseeded and minced

Tempura zucchinis:

1. In a bowl, mix the almond flour, heavy cream, salt, peanut oil, water, and maple syrup.
2. Dredge the zucchini strips in the mixture until well-coated.
3. Heat about 4 tablespoons of olive oil in a non-stick skillet. Working in batches, use tongs to remove the zucchinis (draining extra liquid) into the oil. Fry per side for 1 to 2 minutes and remove the zucchinis onto a paper towel-lined plate to drain grease.
4. Enjoy the zucchinis.

Cream cheese dip:

1. In a bowl, mix the cream cheese, sour cream, taco seasoning, scallion, and green chili.
2. Serve the tempura zucchinis with the cream cheese dip.

TIPS:
Storage: Keep leftovers in the fridge for up to 2 days.
Reheat: Warm zucchinis in the microwave before re-serving.
Serve it with: Add some tempura shrimps to the platter and enjoy more heartily.

NUTRITIONAL FACTS PER SERVING:
Calories: 336 | Total Fat: 34.75g | Carbs: 3.37g
Fiber: 0.2g | Protein 4.16g

Mediterranean Feta and Bacon Skewers

Macros: Fat 80% | Protein 17% | Carbs 3%
Prep time: 15 minutes | Cook time: 8 minutes | Serves: 4

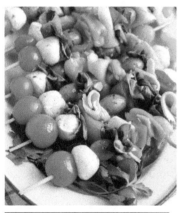

And when you've not had enough of that tasty hummus, add these skewers and possibly, skip lunch. They pair well together as well as serve equally delicious on their own.

2 lb (603 g) feta cheese, cut into 8 cubes
8 bacon slices
4 bamboo skewers, soaked

1 zucchini, cut into 8 bite-size cubes
Salt and black pepper to taste
3 tbsp almond oil for brushing

1. Wrap each feta cube with a bacon slice.
2. Thread one wrapped feta on a skewer; add a zucchini cube, then another wrapped feta, and another zucchini. Repeat the threading process with the remaining skewers.
3. Preheat a grill pan to medium heat, generously brush with the avocado oil and grill the skewer on both sides for 3 to 4 minutes per side or until the set is golden brown and the bacon cooked.
4. Serve afterwards with the tomato salsa.

TIPS:
Storage: Preserve extras in Tupperware and chill for up to 4 days.
Reheat: Warm skewers in the microwave.
Serve it with: Drizzle a blue cheese sauce on the skewers and enjoy for other taste options.

NUTRITIONAL FACTS PER SERVING:
Calories: 753 | Total Fat: 60.05g | carbs: 10.1g | fiber: 0g | protein 43.84g

Cold Avocado & Green Beans Soup

Macros: Fat 89% | Protein 6% | Carbs 5%
Prep time: 15 minutes | Cook time: 11 minutes | Chilling time: 2 hours | Serves: 4

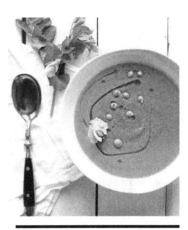

A fantastic way to remind your tummy that lunch or dinner is near. This cold cheesy avo soup also helps in lifting up the fat macros when your mains shortfall of some fatty counts.

1 tbsp butter
2 tbsp almond oil
1 garlic clove, minced
1 cup (227 g) green beans (fresh or frozen)
¼ avocado

1 cup heavy cream
½ cup grated cheddar cheese + extra for garnish
½ tsp coconut aminos
Salt to taste

1. Heat the butter and almond oil in a large skillet and sauté the garlic for 30 seconds. Add the green beans and stir-fry for 10 minutes or until tender.
2. Add the mixture to a food processor and top with the avocado, heavy cream, cheddar cheese, coconut aminos, and salt. Blend the ingredients until smooth.
3. Pour the soup into serving bowls, cover with plastic wraps and chill in the fridge for at least 2 hours.
4. Enjoy afterwards with a garnish of grated white sharp cheddar cheese

TIPS:
Storage: Keep leftovers chilled in the fridge for up to 4 days.
Reheat: None required.
Serve it with: For more flavor, blend some fresh cilantro with the soup and enjoy.

NUTRITIONAL FACTS PER SERVING:
Calories: 301 | Total Fat: 30.34g | Carbs: 4.12g | Fiber: 1.5g | Protein 4.83g

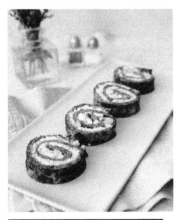

Salmon and Spinach Rolls

Macros: Fat 65% | Protein 32% | Carbs 3%
Prep time: 15 minutes | Cook time: 18 minutes | Serves: 4

These pretty medallion rolls are such a treat! Make them fresh and enjoy them without guilt.

1 1/3 cups (300 g) frozen spinach
1/3 cup (83 g) crumbled mozzarella cheese

3 eggs
3 oz (83 g) smoked salmon
2 cups (454 g) goat cheese

1. Preheat the oven to 400°F/200°C and line a baking tray with a greaseproof paper.
2. Add the spinach to a pot and heat over low heat for 2 to 3 minutes or until wilting. Drain the water off the spinach using a sieve.
3. Crack the eggs onto the spinach, add the mozzarella cheese and mix the ingredients well. Spread the mixture on the baking tray into a large rectangle. Cover with another greaseproof paper and bake in the oven for 15 minutes.
4. Take out the baking tray and remove the top paper. Spread the goat cheese on the spinach and then the smoked salmon. Carefully roll the spinach over the topping into a log.
5. Slice into medallions and enjoy!

TIPS:
Storage: Preserve leftovers in a Tupperware and refrigerate for up to 3 days.
Reheat: None necessary but you may warm the rolls in the microwave as needed.
Serve it with: For improved tastes, drizzle some mayonnaise on the rolls and enjoy.

NUTRITIONAL FACTS PER SERVING:
Calories: 378 | Total Fat: 27.46g | Carbs: 3.12g | Fiber: 1.5g | Protein 29.2g

Supreme Cobb Salad

Macros: Fat 68% | Protein 28% | Carbs 4%
Prep time: 15 minutes | Cook time: 20 minutes | Serves: 4

Wondering why the name "supreme?" Cobb salad naturally includes many elements that makes the salad hefty, which wasn't disputed here. However, the introduction of Parmesan cheese lifts up the fatty requirement of the salad, which improves its taste and flavor to the maximum. You don't find this addition in regular cobb salad.

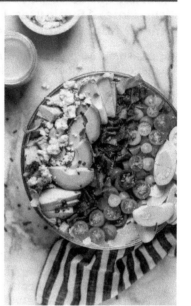

8 bacon slices
1 tbsp olive oil
2 chicken breasts, skin-on and boneless
Salt and black pepper to taste
4 eggs
Ice bath
1 small red onion, chopped
0.5 cup (113.5 g) cherry tomatoes, chopped
0.5 cup (113.5 g) chopped romaine

lettuce
1 cucumber, chopped
1 avocado, chopped
½ cup (113 g) avocado oil
2 tbsp balsamic vinegar
2 tsp Dijon mustard
1 ½ cup (340 g) crumbled blue cheese
2 tbsp grated Parmesan cheese
1 tbsp chopped fresh chives

1. Cook the bacon in a medium non-stick skillet over medium heat on both sides for 2 to 3 minutes per side or until golden brown and crispy. Remove the bacon to a paper towel-lined plate to drain grease. Crumble afterwards.
2. Heat the olive oil in the skillet, season the chicken on both sides with salt, black pepper, and cook in the oil on both sides for 3 to 4 minutes per sides or until golden brown and cooked within. Remove the chicken onto chopping board, rest for 2 minutes and chop the chicken into small cubes.
3. Meanwhile, boil the eggs in about 2 cups of water over medium heat for 7 to 8 minutes. Remove the eggs into the ice bath, let sit for 3 minutes and then peel the eggs. Chop the eggs and place to the side of the chicken.
4. On a serving platter, arrange side by side, the eggs, chicken, onion, tomatoes, lettuce, cucumber, avocado, and sprinkle the bacon on top.
5. In a medium bowl, mix the avocado oil, balsamic vinegar, mustard, and blue cheese. Drizzle the mixture all over the salad and garnish with the Parmesan cheese and chives.
6. Enjoy the salad.

TIPS:
Storage: Keep leftover salad in a bowl, covered and chilled in the fridge for up to 3 days.
Reheat: None required.
Serve it with: Compliment the salad with low-carb bread or fresh berry smoothie.

NUTRITIONAL FACTS PER SERVING:
Calories: 902 | Total Fat: 68.97g | Carbs: 9.91g | Fiber: 2.8g | Protein 60.22g

Creamy Zucchini Soup

Macros: Fat 97% | Protein 1% | Carbs 2%
Prep time: 15 minutes | Cook time: 16 minutes | Serves: 4

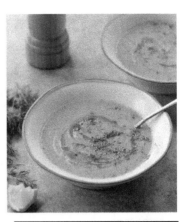

Zucchinis are essential ingredients on the keto diet; however, they could bore you overtime from the frequent faux-pasta use. Try this smooth soup made with zucchinis and some cream as an alternative.

1 tbsp coconut oil
1 medium yellow onion, chopped
3 garlic cloves, minced
4 zucchinis, chopped
2 turnips, peeled and chopped
¼ cup (57 g) chopped fresh cilantro
2 tbsp chopped fresh mint + extra

for garnish
2 tsp curry powder
½ tsp cumin powder
2 cups (454 g) vegetable broth
Salt and black pepper to taste
1 ¼ cups (283 g) almond milk
1 tbsp plain vinegar
¼ tsp red chili flakes

1. Melt the coconut oil in a large pot and sauté the onion for 3 minutes or until softened. Stir in the garlic and cook for 30 seconds or until fragrant.
2. Mix in the zucchinis, turnips, cilantro, mint, curry powder, cumin powder, and vegetable broth. Season with salt, black pepper, and stir well. Bring to a boil and then, simmer for 10 minutes.
3. Use an immersion blender to puree the ingredients until smooth.
4. Stir in the almond milk, vinegar, and simmer for 2 minutes.
5. Dish the soup into serving bowls, garnish with some mint leaves, red chili flakes and serve warm.

TIPS:
Storage: Preserve the soup in a Tupperware and chill in the refrigerator for up to 4 days.
Reheat: Warm in the microwave.
Serve it with: Pair the soup with low-carb bread.

NUTRITIONAL FACTS PER SERVING:
Calories: 653 | Total Fat: 71.84g | Carbs: 4.46g | Fiber: 1.3g | Protein 0.98g

Israeli Salmon Salad

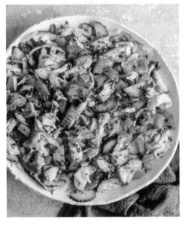

Macros: Fat 70% | Protein 25% | Carbs 5%
Prep time: 5 minutes | Cook time: 0 minutes | Serves: 4

The original salad uses tuna but salmon is one of the best fish to have on the keto diet for its high-fatty composition. Therefore, swapping tuna for smoked salmon excellently worked. Meanwhile, I find that I prefer the taste of salmon in this salad than tuna.

1 cup flaked smoked salmon
1 tomato, chopped
½ small red onion, chopped
1 cucumber, chopped
6 tbsp pitted green olives
1 avocado, chopped
2 tbsp avocado oil

2 tbsp almond oil
1 tbsp plain vinegar
Salt and black pepper to taste
1 cup (227 g) crumbled feta cheese
1 cup (227 g) grated cheddar cheese

TIPS:
Storage: Keep leftover salad in a bowl, covered and chilled in the fridge for up to 3 days.
Reheat: None required.
Serve it with: Enjoy the salad with a chilled glass of homemade cranberry juice.

1. In a salad bowl, add the salmon, tomatoes, red onion, cucumber, green olives, and avocado. Mix well.
2. In a bowl, whisk the avocado oil, vinegar, salt, and black pepper. Drizzle the dressing over the salad and toss well. Top with the feta cheese and serve the salad immediately.

NUTRITIONAL FACTS PER SERVING:
Calories: 636 | Total Fat: 50.65g | Carbs: 8.07g | Fiber: 2.7g | Protein 37.5g

Roasted Tomato and Cheddar Soup

Macros: Fat 79% | Protein 17% | Carbs 4%
Prep time: 10 minutes | Cook time: 15 minutes | Serves: 4

A classic that wins always! I followed the same recipe as we know and touched the top of the soup with some sharp cheddar. Now, this addition is where all the flavor and tastes lies.

2 tbsp butter
2 medium yellow onions, sliced
4 garlic cloves, minced
5 thyme sprigs
8 basil leaves + extra for garnish
8 tomatoes

½ tsp red chili flakes
2 cups (473 g) vegetable broth
Salt and black pepper to taste
1 cup grated cheddar cheese (white and sharp)

1. Melt the butter in a pot and sauté the onions and garlic for 3 minutes or until softened.
2. Stir in the thyme, basil, tomatoes, red chili flakes, and vegetable broth. Season with salt and black pepper.
3. Bring the soup to a boil and then, simmer for 10 minutes or until the tomatoes soften.
4. Use an immersion blender to puree the ingredients until smooth. Adjust the taste with salt and black pepper.
5. Dish the soup into serving bowls and garnish with the cheddar cheese and basil. Serve warm.

TIPS:
Storage: Preserve the soup in a Tupperware and chill in the refrigerator for up to 4 days.
Reheat: Warm in the microwave.
Serve it with: Enjoy the soup with low-carb bread.

NUTRITIONAL FACTS PER SERVING:
Calories: 346 | Total Fat: 30.68g | Carbs: 3.98g | Fiber: 0.8g | Protein 14.5g

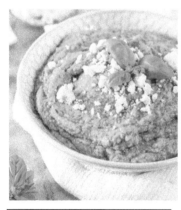

Lemony Avocado Salad with Nutty Pesto

Macros: Fat 82% | Protein 13% | Carbs 4%
Prep time: 10 minutes | Cook time: 0 minutes | Serves: 4

It is tangy, creamy, nutty, and mouthwatering! What good way to introduce nuts into your salad than loading up a pesto with a good handful.

1 cup (227 g) arugula
1 avocado, sliced
½ cup (113 g) cherry tomatoes, halved
3 tbsp plain vinegar, divided
½ cup (118 ml) olive oil
2 tbsp melted butter
10 basil leaves
2 tbsp toasted walnuts

2 tbsp toasted pecans
2 tbsp toasted pine nuts
1 garlic clove, crushed
1 tbsp whole grain mustard
½ cup grated Parmesan cheese
A pinch cayenne pepper
1 tsp xylitol
Salt and black pepper to taste

TIPS:
Storage: Keep leftover salad in a bowl, covered and chilled in the fridge for up to 3 days.
Reheat: None required.
Serve it with: Enjoy the salad with a chilled glass of fresh strawberry juice.

1. In a salad bowl, mix the arugula, avocados, tomatoes, and half of the vinegar.
2. In a food processor, add the olive oil, butter, basil leaves, nuts, garlic, mustard, Parmesan cheese, cayenne pepper, xylitol, salt, and black pepper. Blend at medium speed until the mixture is almost smooth.
3. Drizzle the pesto over the salad, toss well and enjoy!

NUTRITIONAL FACTS PER SERVING:
Calories: 705 | Total Fat: 66.58g | Carbs: 8.01g | Fiber: 4.4g | Protein 22.54g

Spring Salad Mix

Macros: Fat 78% | Protein 19% | Carbs 3%
Prep time: 10 minutes | Cook time: 10 minutes | Serves: 4

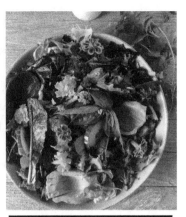

Here's an opportunity to prove that leafy green salads aren't boring. By tossing your favorite leafy greens with mayonnaise, Gruyere cheese and finishing everything off with some bacon, you promise yourself of a good time.

4 oz (113 g) mixed greens
4 tbsp toasted pine nuts
3 tbsp mayonnaise
1 tbsp almond oil

1 cup shaved Gruyere cheese
Salt and black pepper to taste
2 bacon slices, chopped

1. In a bowl, mix the green beans, pine nuts, mayonnaise, almond oil, Gruyere cheese, salt, and black pepper. Set aside for serving.
2. Cook the bacon in a non-stick skillet on both sides for 10 minutes until golden brown and crispy.
3. Sprinkle the bacon on the salad and enjoy!

NUTRITIONAL FACTS PER SERVING:
Calories: 316 | Total Fat: 28.03g | Carbs: 2.69g | Fiber: 1.4g | Protein 14.6g

TIPS:
Storage: Preserve the remaining in the fridge for up to 4 days.
Reheat: None required.
Serve it with: Side the salad to a main dish or enjoy with a low-carb smoothie!

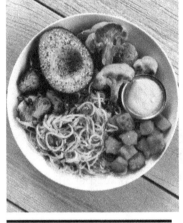

Creamy Tahini Zoodle Soup

Macros: Fat 92% | Protein 3% | Carbs 5%
Prep time: 15 minutes | Cook time: 14 minutes | Serves: 4

Now, you can even make an Asian-inspired noodle soup using zucchinis and tahini. Sounds like an unusual combo? Try it and earn yourself a good opinion.

2 tbsp coconut oil
2 tbsp butter
½ medium onion, chopped
½ cup (113.5 g) sliced cremini mushrooms
1 garlic clove, minced
4 cups (946 g) vegetable broth
4 tbsp coconut aminos
2 tbsp erythritol

2 tbsp tahini
4 tbsp heavy cream
4 zucchinis, spiralized (zoodles)
Topping:
1 tbsp toasted sesame oil for topping
1 tbsp chopped fresh scallions
1 tbsp toasted sesame seeds

TIPS:
Storage: Preserve the soup in a Tupperware and chill in the refrigerator for up to 3 days.
Reheat: Warm in the microwave.
Serve it with: Top the soup with some feta cheese for improved textures.

1. Melt the coconut oil and butter in a pot. Stir-fry the onion, and mushrooms for 5 minutes or until softened. Mix in the garlic and cook for 30 seconds or until fragrant.
2. Add the vegetable broth, coconut aminos, erythritol, tahini, heavy cream, and stir well. Bring the mixture to a boil and then, simmer for 5 minutes.
3. Mix in the zucchinis and cook for 3 minutes or until the zucchinis are tender.
4. Dish the soup into serving bowls and top with the sesame oil, scallions, and sesame seeds.

NUTRITIONAL FACTS PER SERVING:
Calories: 347 | Total Fat: 36.71g | Carbs: 4.47g | Fiber: 1.5g | Protein 2.76g

Creamy Chicken and Mushroom Soup

Macros: Fat 88% | Protein 11% | Carbs 1%
Prep time: 15 minutes | Cook time: 15 minutes | Serves: 4

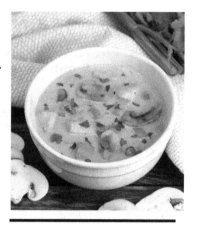

Chicken and mushroom pair well in many dishes because of their identical soft texture. This soup is a creamy blend of both featuring some herbs and spices for a flavor uplift.

1 tbsp olive oil
2 chicken breasts, boneless, with skin
Salt and black pepper to taste
2 cups (454 g) chopped cremini mushrooms
2/3 cup (153 g) chopped onions
1 tsp garlic powder

1 tsp dried parsley
1 tsp turmeric powder
1 tsp paprika
1 cup (237 ml) chicken broth
2 cups (473 ml) almond milk
1 cup (237 ml) heavy cream
½ cup (113 g) grated cheddar cheese (white and sharp)

1. Heat the olive oil in a pot over medium heat, season the chicken with salt, black pepper, and sear in the oil on both sides for 1 minute per side. Remove the chicken onto a plate and set aside.
2. Add the mushrooms, onions, and stir-fry for 5 minutes or until tender. Mix in the garlic powder, parsley, turmeric, and paprika. Cook for 1 minute.
3. Return the chicken to the pot, pour on the chicken broth and stir well. Bring to a boil and then, simmer for 5 to 6 minutes or until the chicken cooks.
4. Use a fork to shred the chicken into strands. Stir in the almond milk, heavy cream, and simmer for 2 minutes and then, adjust the taste with salt and black pepper.
5. Dish the soup into serving bowls, top with the cheddar cheese and serve warm.

TIPS:
Storage: Preserve the soup in a Tupperware and chill in the refrigerator for up to 4 days.
Reheat: Warm in the microwave.
Serve it with: Pair the soup with low-carb bread.

NUTRITIONAL FACTS PER SERVING:
Calories: 1433 | Total Fat: 142.68g | Carbs: 5.04g | Fiber: 1g | Protein 36.06g

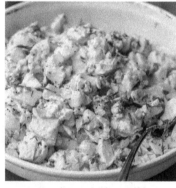

Rich Creamy Egg Salad

Macros: Fat 80% | Protein 19% | Carbs 1%
Prep time: 10 minutes | Cook time: 0 minutes | Serves: 4

This egg salad is one to add to your list of favorite salads because it is rich in taste, nutrients, fattiness, and flavor. It serves well in a sandwich, as a side to a meat dish or enjoyed as itself with any of the drinks shared in the "Drinks" section.

6 eggs
Ice bath
2 tbsp chopped fresh chives
1 tsp Dijon mustard

6 tbsp mayonnaise
2 tbsp sour cream
Salt and black pepper to taste
1 cup finely grated Gruyere cheese

TIPS:
Storage: Keep leftover salad in a bowl, covered and chilled in the fridge for up to 2 days.
Reheat: None required.
Serve it with: You may also enjoy the salad in a sandwich using low-carb bread slices.

1. Boil the eggs in about 2 cups of water over medium heat for 7 to 8 minutes. Remove the eggs into the ice bath, let sit for 3 minutes and then peel the eggs. Chop the eggs and add to a salad mixing bowl.
2. Top with the chives, Dijon mustard, mayonnaise, sour cream, salt, black pepper, and Gruyere cheese. Mix well and serve immediately.

NUTRITIONAL FACTS PER SERVING:
Calories: 374 | Total Fat: 33.33g | Carbs: 1.04g | Fiber: 0.1g | Protein 16.79g

Salad Nicoise with a Twist

Macros: Fat 75% | Protein 23% | Carbs 3%
Prep time: 18 minutes | Cook time: 28 minutes | Serves: 4

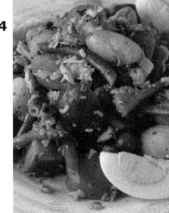

Take out the potatoes in the classic Nicoise salad and replace it with turnips for a keto-safe option. You'll love this one!

½ cup (113.5 g) peeled and quartered turnips
¼ cup (57 g) green beans
½ cup olive oil
Salt and black pepper to taste
4 eggs
2 tbsp grainy mustard

2 lemons, juiced
2 garlic cloves, minced
1 (10.5 oz) can (300 g) tuna flakes, drained
1 tbsp chopped fresh parsley
¼ cup grated Gruyere cheese

1. Preheat the oven to 400°F/200°C and grease a baking tray with olive oil.
2. Add the turnips and green beans. Drizzle with 1 tablespoon of olive oil and season with salt and black pepper. Use your hands to massage the seasoning on the vegetables. Bake in the oven for 20 minutes or until the turnips soften and the green beans are slightly charred.
3. Meanwhile, boil the eggs in a pot of water for 7 to 8 minutes. Afterwards, transfer the eggs to an ice bath, let cool for 3 minutes, and then peel the eggs. Slice in halves and set aside on a plate.
4. In a bowl, make the dressing; whisk the mustard, vinegar, garlic, and remaining olive oil.
5. On a serving platter, spread the turnips and green beans. Add the tuna, parsley, and eggs. Drizzle the dressing on top, garnish with the Parmesan cheese, and serve immediately.

TIPS:
Storage: Preserve extra salad in a plastic bowls and chill in the refrigerator for up to 3 days.
Reheat: None required.
Serve it with: For a fuller serve, enjoy with steamed cauliflower rice.

NUTRITIONAL FACTS PER SERVING:
Calories: 410 | Total Fat: 34.7g | Carbs: 2.86g | Fiber: 0.8g | Protein 22.69g

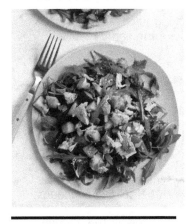

Greek Tuna Salad

Macros: Fat 65% | Protein 30% | Carbs 5%
Prep time: 10 minutes | Cook time: 0 minutes | Serves: 4

Do you remember the Israeli Salmon Salad we made earlier? This salad is where I threw all that tuna. Now, combining Greek yogurt with flaked tuna and some flavorful vegetables is what I call a winning reconstruction. Enjoy the terrific taste!

3 (5 oz) (425 g) cans tuna in water, drained and flaked
¼ small red onion, finely chopped
1 celery stalks, finely chopped
½ avocado, chopped
1 tbsp chopped fresh parsley

1 cup (227 g) Greek yogurt
2 tbsp butter
2 tsp Dijon Mustard
½ tbsp vinegar
Salt and black pepper to taste

1. Add all the ingredients to a salad bowl and mix until well combined.
2. Serve afterwards.

TIPS:
Storage: Refrigerate leftovers for up to a week.
Reheat: None required.
Serve it with: Fill up a low-carb sandwich with the salad or serve with fried chicken.

NUTRITIONAL FACTS PER SERVING:
Calories: 292 | Total Fat: 21.67g | Carbs: 4.13g | Fiber: 2g | Protein 22.09g

Creamy Seafood Soup

Macros: Fat 80% | Protein 15% | Carbs 5%
Prep time: 10 minutes | Cook time: 5 minutes | Serves: 4

I tried a Spanish seafood mix at my best friend, Lucy's house once. I was blown away by the flavor that exuded from the blend of different seafood. Of course, I tried it, kicked in some cooking cream and couldn't be more grateful for that experience. Here is my share with you.

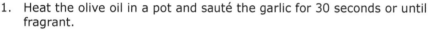

1 tbsp avocado oil
2 garlic cloves, minced
¾ tbsp almond flour
1 cup (236 ml) vegetable broth
1 tsp dried dill

1 lb (454 g) frozen mixed seafood
Salt and black pepper to taste
1 tbsp plain vinegar
2 cups (454 g) cooking cream
Fresh dill leaves to garnish

1. Heat the olive oil in a pot and sauté the garlic for 30 seconds or until fragrant.
2. Stir in the almond flour until brown.
3. Mix in the vegetable broth until smooth and stir in the dill, seafood mix, salt, and black pepper. Bring the soup to a boil and then simmer for 3 to 4 minutes or until the seafood cooks.
4. Add the vinegar, cooking cream and stir well.
5. Dish the soup into serving bowls, garnish with fresh dill and serve warm.

NUTRITIONAL FACTS PER SERVING:
Calories: 401 | Total Fat: 36.6g | Carbs: 5.18g | Fiber: 0.1g | Protein 14.82g

TIPS:
Storage: Preserve the soup in a Tupperware and chill in the refrigerator for up to 4 days.
Reheat: Warm in the microwave.
Serve it with: Pair the soup with low-carb bread.

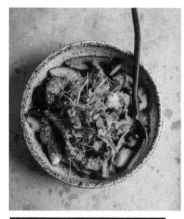

Super Green Bowl Salad

Macros: Fat 72% | Protein 23% | Carbs 5%
Prep time: 15 minutes | Cook time: 8 minutes | Serves: 4

Cleaning the gut doesn't require only a detoxing juice. A salad that sits all the right ingredients would help you achieve the same results. For weight loss, I highly recommend this salad.

2 broccoli heads, cut into florets
½ avocado, sliced and divided
1 cup (227 g) baby spinach
1 cucumber, chopped
1 tbsp plain vinegar
2 tbsp chopped fresh cilantro

2 tsp sugar-free maple syrup
½ cup (113 g) water
Salt and black pepper to taste
1 cup grated cheddar cheese (white and sharp)
1 cup crumbled goat cheese

TIPS:
Storage: Keep leftover salad in a bowl, covered and chilled in the fridge for up to 3 days.
Reheat: None required.
Serve it with: A good glass of water will wash down this salad just good!

1. Soften the broccoli in a steamer for 5 to 8 minutes. Remove the vegetables into a serving bowl and top with half of the avocados, spinach, and cucumber.
2. In a bowl, mash the remaining avocados and mix in the vinegar, cilantro, maple syrup, water, salt, and black pepper until well-combined.
3. Drizzle the avocado dressing on the salad, top with the cheddar cheese, goat cheese and serve immediately.

NUTRITIONAL FACTS PER SERVING:
Calories: 344 | Total Fat: 28.12g | Carbs: 4.52g | Fiber: 2.3g | Protein 19.46g

Chicken Schnitzel with Asparagus

Macros: Fat 78% | Protein 21% | Carbs 1%
Prep time: 15 minutes | Cook time: 16 minutes | Serves: 4

You've eaten chicken many times in your life, why not try something different for the next one? Crusting chicken with ground nuts and cheese is the way to go! Unlike a breadcrumb crusted chicken, these pieces sit on top a hefty, crunchy goodness of healthy fats.

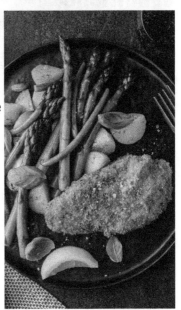

1 tbsp chopped fresh parsley
4 garlic cloves, minced
1 tbsp plain vinegar
1 tbsp coconut aminos
2 tsp sugar-free maple syrup
2 tsp chili pepper
Salt and black pepper to taste
6 tbsp coconut oil
1 lb (680 g) asparagus, hard stems removed

4 chicken breasts, skin-on and boneless
2 cups (240 g) grated Mexican cheese blend
1 tbsp mixed sesame seeds
1 cup (120 g) almond flour
4 eggs, beaten
6 tbsp avocado oil
1 tsp chili flakes for garnish

1. In a bowl, whisk the parsley, garlic, vinegar, coconut aminos, maple syrup, chili pepper, salt, and black pepper. Set aside.
2. Heat the coconut oil in a large skillet and stir-fry the asparagus for 8 to 10 minutes or until tender. Remove the asparagus into a large bowl and toss with the vinegar mixture. Set aside for serving.
3. Cover the chicken breasts in plastic wraps and use a meat tenderizer to gently pound the chicken until flattened to 2-inch thickness.
4. On a plate, mix the Mexican cheese blend and sesame seeds. Dredge the chicken pieces in the almond flour, dip in the egg on both sides, and generously coat in the seed mix.
5. Heat the avocado oil in a large skillet over medium heat. Cook the chicken for 3 minutes per side or until golden brown and cooked within.
6. Divide the asparagus onto 4 serving plates, place a chicken on each, and garnish with the chili flakes. Serve warm.

TIPS:
Storage: Keep the chicken and asparagus in separate Tupperwares and refrigerate for up to 4 days.
Reheat: Warm both chicken and asparagus in the microwave.
Serve it with: Include a sweet cheese sauce with the dish for improved tastes.

NUTRITIONAL FACTS PER SERVING:
Calories: 1541 | Total Fat: 136.26g | Carbs: 5.58g | Fiber: 2.7g | Protein 75.51g

Tomato Soup with Grilled Cheese Sandwiches

Macros: Fat 78% | Protein 18% | Carbs 4%
Prep time: 18 minutes | Cook time: 38 minutes | Serves: 4

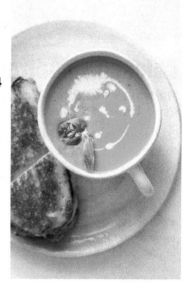

It comes across as a light meal and may question its ability to satisfy fully. Well, the cheese stuffed sandwiches make up for the quantity that your tummy needs for a fill. And if you're feeling spicy, kick up the soup with some red chilies.

3 tbsp unsalted butter, divided
1 tbsp almond oil
1 (7 oz) (198 g) cans crushed tomatoes
2 medium white onions, chopped
1 ½ cups water
Salt and black pepper to taste

1 tsp dried basil
8 low-carb bread slices
1 cup (227 g) Gruyere cheese
½ cup (113.5 g) grated Monterey Jack cheese
1 tbsp chopped fresh basil for garnish

1. Melt 2 tablespoons of butter in a pot and mix in the tomatoes, onions, and water. Season with salt, black pepper, basil, and bring the mixture to a boil. Reduce the heat immediately and simmer for 30 minutes or until the liquid reduces by a third.
2. Meanwhile, melt a ¼ tablespoon of butter in a non-stick skillet over medium heat and lay in a bread slice.
3. Add a quarter each of both cheese on top and cover with another bread slice. Once the cheese starts melting and beneath the bread is golden brown, about 1 minute, flip the sandwich. Cook further for 1 more minute or until the other side of the bread is golden brown too.
4. Remove the sandwich to a plate and make three more in the same manner. Afterwards, diagonally slice each sandwich in half.
5. Dish the tomato soup into serving bowls when ready, garnish with the basil leaves, and serve warm with the sandwiches.

TIPS:
Storage: Refrigerate remaining soup in plastic bowls with covers. Wrap the sandwiches in greaseproof paper and chill in the refrigerator for up to 4 days.
Reheat: Warm both soup and sandwiches in the microwave before re-enjoying.
Serve it with: For a thicker soup, whisk in some heavy cream when the soup is about 2 minutes away from being done.

NUTRITIONAL FACTS PER SERVING:
Calories: 285 | Total Fat: 25.2g | Carbs: 3.41g | Fiber: 1.3g | Protein 12.22g

Steak and Green Beans with Coconut Tarragon Sauce

Macros: Fat 69% | Protein 28% | Carbs 3%
Prep time: 15 minutes | Cook time: 25 minutes | Serves: 4

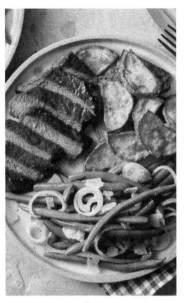

Steak with green beans or asparagus is regular for lunch but not the flavor-bursting tarragon sauce that it comes with. If you're thinking of where most of the keto fat elements lie, don't ignore the sauce. It is nutritious and makes the entire dish shine.

2 tbsp olive oil
2 tbsp almond oil
4 (900 g) beef entrecote
Salt and black pepper to taste
1 cup (227 g) green beans
1 cup (227 g) small whole tomatoes
½ shallot chopped

2 garlic cloves, minced
2/3 cup (150 ml) white wine
2 cups (400 ml) coconut cream
4 tbsp unsalted butter
¼ cup chopped fresh tarragon + extra for garnish
1 tsp freshly squeezed vinegar
Flaky sea salt for garnish

1. Heat the olive oil and almond oil in a large skillet over medium heat and cook the beef for 10 to 15 minutes or until brown and cooked within. Remove the beef onto a plate and set aside covered with foil.
2. Add the green beans and tomatoes to the pot. Stir-fry for 5 to 7 minutes or until the vegetables soften. Remove onto a plate and cover.
3. Sauté the shallots and garlic in the skillet for 1 minute and deglaze the pan with the white wine.
4. Whisk in the coconut cream and butter until the butter melts. Stir in the tarragon, vinegar, and season with salt and black pepper. Simmer for 1 to 2 minutes and turn the heat off.
5. Make 4 beds of the green beans on 4 plates, top with a steak each, side with the tomatoes, and drizzle the tarragon sauce on top. Garnish with more tarragon, flaky salt, and serve immediately!

TIPS:
Storage: Refrigerate remaining beef, green beans, and tomatoes in a Tupperware for up to 4 days.
Reheat: Warm food in the microwave.
Serve it with: Increase the portion size with mashed cauliflower or turnips.

NUTRITIONAL FACTS PER SERVING:
Calories: 735 | Total Fat: 57.61g | Carbs: 5.85g | Fiber: 1.2g | Protein 51.17g

Yogurt Loaded Smashed Turnips

Macros: Fat 89% | Protein 7% | Carbs 4%
Prep time: 20 minutes | Cook time: 42 minutes | Serves: 4

Comfort foods or familiar foods is one way to reach success on the keto diet. By swapping ingredients in a particular food to suit the diet, meal preps become an easy task. That's what I do with this idea; using the familiar smashed potato recipe that we know and using turnips instead. Then, I made sure to load it up with seasoned full-fat yogurt for a good taste.

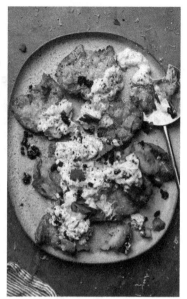

½ lb (227 g) turnips
1/3 cup (78 ml) avocado oil
Salt and black pepper to taste
1 cup (237 g) full-fat Greek yogurt
1 red onion, finely chopped
¾ cup (181 g) chopped fresh cilantro + extra for garnish

1/3 cup (74 g) chopped fresh mint + extra for garnish
2 tsp sugar-free maple syrup
½ lemon, juiced
1 cup (227 g) chopped cheddar cheese (white and sharp)
2 tbsp chopped toasted almonds

1. Preheat the oven to 400°F/200°C.
2. Add the turnips and 2 to 3 cups of salted water to a pot. Cook the turnips for 10 to 12 minutes or until a fork inserted into the turnips comes out clean. Drain the turnips and pat dry with a paper towel.
3. Add the turnips to a baking tray and use the bottom of a glass bottle to smash the turnips. Drizzle with the avocado oil and season with salt and black pepper. Bake in the oven for 30 minutes or until golden brown and crispy, flipping halfway.
4. In a medium bowl, mix the Greek yogurt with the onion, cilantro, mint, maple syrup, and vinegar.
5. When the turnips are ready, remove from the oven and immediately sprinkle with the cheddar cheese.
6. Dish the food onto serving plates and top with the yogurt mixture. Add the almonds and garnish with some cilantro and mint. Enjoy immediately!

TIPS:
Storage: Add extra turnips to a Tupperware and refrigerate for up to 4 days. Also, keep the yogurt topping sauce covered in the refrigerator for the same period.
Reheat: Warm the turnips in the microwave and serve with the yogurt topping sauce.
Serve it with: Swap the cheddar cheese for goat or feta cheese for a more Mediterranean feel.

NUTRITIONAL FACTS PER SERVING:
Calories: 546 | Total Fat: 54.95g | Carbs: 5.66g | Fiber: 2g | Protein 9.27g

Creamy Pork and Celeriac Gratin

Macros: Fat 77% | Protein 19% | Carbs 4%
Prep time: 20 minutes | Cook time: 1 hour 8 minutes |
Serves: 4

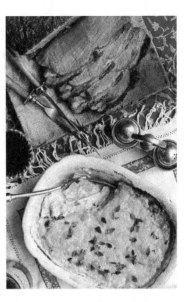

I love one-dish bakes just like this gratin. I chose to use pork for the intense meat aroma but you may use other meat types like beef, lamb, or chicken.

½ lb celeriac, peeled and thinly sliced
1/3 cup almond milk
½ cup heavy cream
¼ tsp nutmeg powder
Salt and black pepper to taste
1 tbsp olive oil
1 lb ground pork

½ medium white onion, chopped
1 garlic clove, minced
½ tsp unsweetened tomato paste
3 tbsp butter for greasing
1 cup (227 g) crumbled quesco fresco cheese
1 tbsp chopped fresh parsley for garnish

1. Preheat the oven to 350°F/180°C.
2. In a saucepan, add the celeriac, almond milk, heavy cream, nutmeg powder, and salt. Cook over medium heat for 7 to 9 minutes or until the celeriac softens. Drain afterwards and set aside.
3. Meanwhile, heat the olive oil in a skillet and cook the pork for 5 minutes or until starting to brown. Season with salt and black pepper.
4. Stir in the onion, garlic, and cook for 5 minutes or until the onions soften. Mix in the tomato paste and cook for 2 to 3 minutes.
5. Grease a baking dish with butter and layer half of the celeriac on the bottom of the dish. Spread the tomato-pork sauce on top and cover with the remaining celeriac. Finish the topping with the queso fresco cheese.
6. Bake in the oven for 40 to 45 minutes or until the cheese melts and is golden brown. Remove from the oven to cool for 5 to 10 minutes, garnish with the parsley, and serve afterwards.

TIPS:
Storage: Preserve remaining food in a Tupperware and refrigerate for up to 4 days.
Reheat: Warm gratin in microwave.
Serve it with: Add more texture to the dish with coconut oil-sautéed cremini mushrooms or green beans.

NUTRITIONAL FACTS PER SERVING:
Calories: 785 | Total Fat: 67.52g | Carbs: 8.34g | Fiber: 1.4g | Protein 36.1g

Gruyere Chicken in Tomato Sauce

Macros: Fat 61% | Protein 36% | Carbs 2%
Prep time: 15 minutes | Cook time: 16 minutes | Serves: 4

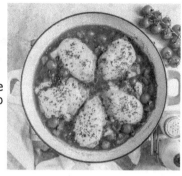

The original of this recipe is Parmesan chicken but isn't Parmesan cheese with chicken overrated? For a change, introduce some Gruyere cheese to the dish and change things up entirely.

2 tbsp olive oil
½ large yellow onion
2 garlic cloves, minced
1 tsp dried basil
1 (7 oz) unsweetened tomato sauce
Salt and black pepper to taste

4 chicken breasts, skin-on and boneless
1 cup (227 g) grated Gruyere cheese + extra for serving
1 ½ cup (340 g) pork rinds
2 eggs, beaten

1. Heat the olive oil in a pot and sauté the onion for 3 minutes or until tender. Stir in the garlic, basil, and cook for 30 seconds or until fragrant.
2. Mix in the tomato sauce, cover the lid and simmer for 8 to 10 minutes or until the sauce thickens. Season with salt and black pepper.
3. Season the chicken with salt and black pepper. In a bowl, mix the Gruyere cheese and pork rinds. Dip the chicken in the eggs and generously coat in the cheese mix.
4. Heat the remaining olive oil in a skillet over medium heat and fry the chicken on both sides for 2 to 3 minutes per side or until golden brown and cooked within.
5. Spoon the tomato sauce onto dip serving plates, top with the chicken, more Gruyere cheese and enjoy!

TIPS:
Storage: Refrigerate chicken and tomato sauce into two separate bowls for up to 3 days.
Reheat: Warm both chicken and sauce in the microwave.
Serve it with: Enjoy better with creamy mashed parsnips or sautéed green beans.

NUTRITIONAL FACTS PER SERVING:
Calories : 959 | Total Fat: 65.82g | Carbs: 5.77g | Fiber: 1.2g | Protein 82.34g

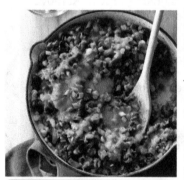

Chili Taco Skillet

Macros: Fat 76% | Protein 19% | Carbs 5%
Prep time: 15 minutes | Cook time: 26 minutes | Serves: 4

The taco idea is trending in many dishes; soups, bakes, snacks, and many more. Why not get onto the fun ride and make this skillet loaded meal flavored with taco seasoning?

2 tbsp avocado oil
2 tbsp almond oil
½ lb (250 g) ground beef
½ medium red bell pepper
½ large yellow onion
1 red chili, minced
2 tbsp taco seasoning
Topping:
1 cup sour cream
½ avocado, chopped

1 (7 oz) (200 g) can diced tomatoes
Salt and black pepper to taste
1 cup (150 g) baby kale
1 ½ cups (200 g) grated cheddar cheese (white and sharp)

1 tbsp chopped fresh scallions

TIPS:
Storage: Preserve remaining food in a Tupperware and refrigerate for up to 5 days.
Reheat: Warm in the microwave.
Serve it with: Serve with low-carb tortilla chips, cauliflower rice, or zucchini chips.

NUTRITIONAL FACTS PER SERVING:
Calories: 580 | Total Fat: 49.44g | Carbs: 8.01g | Fiber: 3.4g | Protein 27.31g

1. Heat the avocado oil in a skillet and cook the beef for 5 minutes or until starting to brown.
2. Stir in the bell peppers, onion, red chili, and taco seasoning. Cook for 5 minutes or until the vegetables soften.
3. Mix in the tomatoes, cover the lid, and cook for 10 minutes or until the tomatoes become tender.
4. Season with salt, black pepper, and stir in the kale. Cook for 2 to 3 minutes or until the kale wilts.
5. Mix in the cheddar cheese, let melt for 2 to 3 minutes, and turn the heat off.
6. Dish the food onto serving plates and top with the sour cream, avocado, and scallions. Serve immediately.

Zoodle Alla Cabonara

Macros: Fat 83% | Protein 13% | Carbs 4%
Prep time: 15 minutes | Cook time: 18 minutes | Serves: 4

Yes! We can have carbonara on the keto diet. A faux one with zoodles that happens to be tastier than the original.

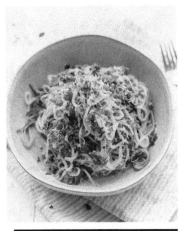

8 bacon slices, chopped
3 tbsp butter
1 cup (227 g) chopped cremini mushrooms
½ medium yellow onion, chopped
1 cup (227 g) heavy cream

2 cups (454 g) zoodles, spiralized zucchinis
Salt and black pepper to taste
1 cup (227 g) grated Gruyere cheese
Fresh basil leaves for garnish

1. Cook the bacon in a large skillet for 8 to 10 minutes or until brown and crispy. Remove onto a paper towel-lined plate to drain grease and set aside.
2. Melt the butter in the skillet and stir-fry the mushrooms and onion for 5 minutes or until softened.
3. Stir in the heavy cream; once starts boiling, mix in the zucchinis and season with salt and black pepper. Cook for 2 to 3 minutes or until the zucchinis are fork tender.
4. Stir in the bacon and Gruyere cheese. Dish the food, garnish with basil leaves and serve warm.

TIPS:
Storage: Keep remaining food in a Tupperware and chill for up to 3 days.
Reheat: Warm the food in microwave.
Serve it with: Top with the dish with sunshine-fried eggs.

NUTRITIONAL FACTS PER SERVING:
Calories: 523 | Total Fat: 49.17g | Carbs: 5.2g | Fiber: 1g | Protein 16.85g

Italian Cauliflower and Sausage Bowl

Macros: Fat 81% | Protein 15% | Carbs 4%
Prep time: 12 minutes | Cook time: 16 minutes | Serves: 4

Making veggies and meat bowls is easy, straightforward and comfortable to have. This dish cooks in little time, which makes it a go-to when the hunger pangs surprisingly set in.

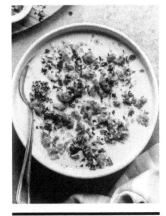

TIPS:
Storage: Keep the remaining food in a Tupperware and chill for up to 3 days.
Reheat: Warm the food in the microwave.
Serve it with: For more excitement, introduce a blend of cheese for topping and enjoy the dish with fresh berry juice.

¼ cup olive oil
7 oz Italian sausages, sliced into 1-inch rings
½ small head cauliflower, cut into florets
1 large zucchini, chopped
1 garlic clove, minced

1 tsp red chili flakes
1 tbsp plain vinegar
Salt and black pepper to taste
1 ½ cups grated Gruyere cheese
1 tbsp chopped fresh basil for garnish

1. Heat the olive oil in large frying pan and cook the sausages on both sides until golden brown, 5 minutes. Remove the sausages onto a paper towel-lined plate to drain grease and set aside.
2. Add the cauliflower to the skillet and cook until softened, 5 minutes. Stir in the zucchini, cook for 3 minutes and introduce the garlic. Mix and let the fragrance release for 30 seconds. Season with the red chili flakes, vinegar, salt, and black pepper.
3. Return the sausages to the skillet, stir well, and simmer for 1 to 2 minutes.
4. Dish the food onto serving plates, top with the Gruyere cheese, and garnish with the basil. Serve immediately.

NUTRITIONAL FACTS PER SERVING:
Calories: 661 | Total Fat: 61.3g | Carbs: 6.83g | Fiber: 2.1g | Protein 24.7g

Lamb Stuffed Bell Peppers

Macros: Fat 79% | Protein 16% | Carbs 5%
Prep time: 15 minutes | Cook time: 38 minutes | Serves: 4

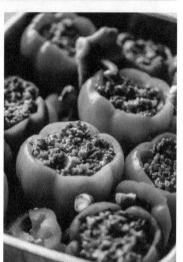

I love the idea of not including bell peppers in meatballs but instead filling bell peppers with meat before baking them. The flavor of the sweet peppers infuses the meat well for a delicious treat.

½ lb (¼ kg) ground lamb
½ medium yellow onions, chopped
2 garlic cloves, minced
4 tbsp toasted almonds, finely chopped
1 tsp dried parsley
½ tsp dried marjoram
1 tsp paprika
1 tbsp mustard
1 egg

2 cups (454 g) grated cheddar cheese
Salt and black pepper to taste
4 large red bell peppers, halved and deseeded
4 tbsp almond oil
1 tbsp unsweetened tomato paste
2/3 cup (200 ml) red wine
1 1/3 cup (333 ml) vegetable broth

1. Preheat the oven to 320°F/160°C.
2. In a bowl, add the lamb, half of the onions, garlic, almonds, parsley, marjoram, paprika, mustard, egg, cheddar cheese, salt, and black pepper. Mix well and divide the mixture into the bell peppers. Fit in well and level the top flat.
3. Heat the almond oil in an oven-proof pot over medium heat, add the peppers, and brown on all sides for 2 minutes per side. Remove the peppers onto a plate and set aside.
4. Sauté the remaining onions in the pot and stir in the tomato paste. Deglaze the pan with the red wine and cook for 1 minute or until the red wine reduces by half. Mix in the vegetable broth and return the peppers to the pot with meat side up.
5. Cover the pot and bake in the oven for 30 minutes or until the peppers soften and the sauce reduced.
6. Remove the pot and dish the food. Garnish with the parsley and serve warm.

TIPS:
Storage: Keep leftovers in a Tupperware and refrigerate for up to 4 days.
Reheat: Warm food in microwave before serving.
Serve it with: Enjoy best with herby cauliflower rice.

NUTRITIONAL FACTS PER SERVING:
Calories: 617 | Total Fat: 54.56g | Carbs: 8.56g | Fiber: 2.4g | Protein 24.41g

Braised Steak in Creamy Vinegar Sauce

Macros: Fat 71% | Protein 25% | Carbs 4%
Prep time: 15 minutes | Cook time: 21 minutes | Serves: 4

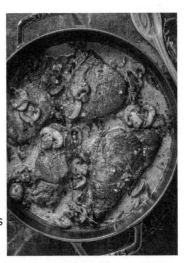

You'll love this quick combination when you're running late to serve dinner. Meanwhile, it is a pretty, healthy look that will get the family drooling for a dig in.

Braised steak:

½ lb (¼ kg) beef round roast
Salt and black pepper to taste
1 tbsp almond flour
4 ½ tbsp butter
1 small white onion
1 garlic clove, minced
2 celery stalks, chopped

1 bay leaf
¼ cup (59 ml) white wine vinegar
1 cup (237 ml) beef stock
½ cup (118 ml) heavy cream
½ cup (114 g) green beans, strings removed
1 tbsp swerve sugar

1. Season the beef on both sides with salt, black pepper, and dust with the almond flour.
2. Melt 3 ½ tablespoons of butter in a wide pot and sauté the onion for 5 to 6 minutes or until browning. Put the beef in the pot and sear on both sides for 4 to 5 minutes per side or until golden brown.
3. Add the garlic, celery, and bay leaf. Cook for 1 minute and pour in the vinegar. Let the vinegar evaporate for about 1 minute.
4. Pour the beef stock into the pan to deglaze the bottom. Cover the pot, reduce the heat to low and simmer for 3 minutes.
5. After, remove the beef onto a chopping board and set aside while you finish the sauce.
6. Stir the heavy cream into the sauce until well combined, then strain the sauce and return to the pot. Season with salt and black pepper.
7. Slice the beef into small pieces, return to the sauce and stir well. Simmer for 1 minute and turn the heat off.
8. Melt the remaining butter in a skillet, add the green beans and season with the swerve sugar and some salt. Stir-fry for 5 minutes or until the green beans are fork-tender.
9. Dish the beef with sauce and green beans. Serve immediately.

TIPS:
Storage: Preserve leftovers in a separate bowl and chill for up to 3 days.
Reheat: Warm both beef and sauce, and green beans in the microwave.
Serve it with: Pair the dish with creamy mashed cauliflower.

NUTRITIONAL FACTS PER SERVING:
Calories: 305 | Total Fat: 24.56g | Carbs: 3.39g | Fiber: 0.8g | Protein 17.77g

Swedish Pork Meatballs

Macros: Fat 86% | Protein 13% | Carbs 1%
Prep time: 20 minutes | Cook time: 23 minutes | Serves: 4

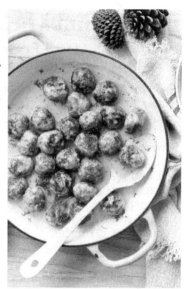

The classic Swedish meatballs earns its place here for its winning taste but with slight changes - pork instead of beef, low-carb bread instead of regular bread, and some pork rinds for firming the meatballs instead of Panko breadcrumbs.

½ cup (100 ml) almond milk
1 low-carb bread loaf, cut into small cubes
3 tbsp olive oil for frying
1 medium onion, finely chopped
½ lb (¼ kg) ground pork
1 egg
2 tbsp crushed pork rinds
Salt and black pepper to taste

1 tbsp butter
1 tbsp almond flour
1 ¼ cup (300 ml) chicken stock
½ cup (120 ml) heavy cream
1 tsp allspice powder
2 tsp coconut aminos
1 tbsp chopped fresh scallions for garnish

1. Add the almond milk and bread to a bowl. Let the bread soak while you sauté the onions.
2. Heat 1 tsp of olive oil in a skillet over medium heat and stir-fry the onions for 3 minutes or until translucent.
3. Pour the onions into the bread bowl and add the pork, egg, pork rinds, salt, and black pepper. Mix well and form 1-inch meatballs from the mixture.
4. Heat the remaining olive oil in the skillet and fry the meatballs on both sides for 3 to 4 minutes per side or until golden brown, and cooked within. Remove the meatballs onto a plate and set aside.
5. Melt the butter in the skillet and sauté the almond flour until browning and stir in the chicken stock.
6. Whisk in the heavy cream and simmer for 5 to 7 minutes or until the sauce thickens. Season with the allspice powder, coconut aminos, salt (as needed), and black pepper.
7. Return the meatballs to the skillet, baste with the sauce, and simmer for 30 seconds. Turn the heat off.
8. Garnish with the scallions and serve the food immediately.

TIPS:
Storage: Refrigerate the remaining meatballs with sauce in a Tupperware and keep for up to 3 days.
Reheat: Warm food in the microwave.
Serve it with: Top the food with homemade (low-carb) raspberry jam and serve with mashed turnips.

NUTRITIONAL FACTS PER SERVING:
Calories: 911 | Total Fat: 87.73g | Carbs: 3.52g | Fiber: 0.6g | Protein 27.18g

Peruvian Chicken Roast with Creamy Green Sauce

Macros: Fat 68% | Protein 30% | Carbs 2%
Prep time: 20 minutes | Cook time: 50 minutes | Serves: 4

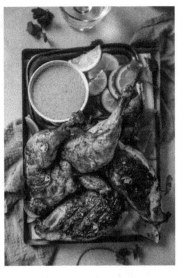

I took a cooking class while visiting Peru and this dish was the first one I made. The name may sound intimidating but it is a straightforward make. It is a regular chicken roast with slight changes in seasoning. Meanwhile, don't miss out the complimenting green sauce. It brings on a worth of flavor to the plate.

Peruvian Chicken:

1 (4 lb) (1814 g) whole chicken, butterflied
4 tsp salt
1 ½ tbsp smoked paprika
1 ½ tbsp cumin powder
1 tsp dried oregano
1 tsp black peppercorns, crushed
3 garlic cloves, minced
4 tbsp olive oil + extra for brushing
3 tbsp white vinegar

Creamy Green Sauce:

2 green chili peppers
½ cup fresh cilantro leaves
1 tsp plain vinegar
2 garlic cloves, minced
2 tbsp avocado oil
Salt and black pepper to taste
½ cup (118 ml) mayonnaise
½ cup (118 ml) heavy cream

Peruvian chicken:

1. Preheat the oven to 400°F/200°C and brush a baking tray with olive oil.
2. Pat the chicken dry with paper towel and lay on the baking tray.
3. In a bowl, mix the salt, paprika, cumin powder, oregano, black peppercorns, garlic, olive oil, and vinegar. Brush the mixture all over the chicken, in and out.
4. Roast the chicken in the oven for 10 minutes. Reduce the temperature to 320°F/160°C and brush the chicken with the juices in the pan. Roast further for 40 minutes or until the chicken fully cooks.
5. Remove the tray afterwards and let the chicken rest for 10 minutes before slicing.
6. Meanwhile, make the creamy green sauce.
7. In a food processor, add the green chili peppers, cilantro, vinegar, garlic, and avocado oil. Blend until almost smooth. Season with salt, black pepper, and pour in the mayonnaise and heavy cream. Process again until well combined.
8. Dish the sliced chicken and serve with the creamy green sauce.

TIPS:
Storage: Keep leftovers of both chicken, and sauce in plastic bowls and refrigerate for up to a week.
Reheat: Warm the chicken in the microwave and serve straightaway with the green sauce.
Serve it with: Add some parsnip fries to the platter and enjoy heartily. You may also swap heavy cream for sour cream. Make sure to make plenty of sauce too because it runs out fast.

NUTRITIONAL FACTS PER SERVING:
Calories: 709 | Total Fat: 53.96g | Carbs: 5.19g | Fiber: 1.3g | Protein 50.12g

Indian Chicken Coconut Curry

Macros: Fat 80% | Protein 17% | Carbs 3%
Prep time: 15 minutes | Cook time: 32 minutes | Serves: 4

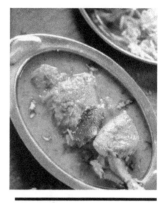

Making Indian curries may be intimidating, so I made a simple and straightforward version for quick dinner fixes. Enjoy it with cauliflower rice or mashed turnips.

4 tbsp coconut oil
2 (250 g) chicken breasts, cut into bite-size cubes
Salt and black pepper to taste
1 (8 oz) (227 g) pack paneer cheese, cut into bite-size cubes
1 tbsp fresh ginger paste
1 tbsp garam masala
1 medium red bell pepper, deseeded and chopped
½ medium red onion, chopped
1 (7 oz) can tomato sauce
1 cup (200 ml) almond milk
2 lemongrass sticks, chopped
2 tbsp chopped fresh cilantro + extra to garnish
2 heaping tsp red curry paste
¼ tsp turmeric

1. Melt the coconut oil in a pot over medium heat, season the chicken with salt, black pepper, and sear in the oil for 2 minutes per side or until golden brown. Remove the chicken onto a plate and set aside.
2. Sear the paneer cheese in the oil for 1 minute per side or until golden brown. Remove to the side of the chicken.
3. Add the ginger and garam masala to the oil, and stir-fry for 1 to 2 minutes or until the flavor releases.
4. Stir in the bell peppers and onions; cook for 3 minutes or until tender.
5. Pour in the tomato sauce, almond milk, lemongrass, cilantro, curry paste, and turmeric. Stir well, cover, bring to a boil, and then simmer for 10 minutes.
6. Return the chicken and paneer cheese to the pot and continue cooking simmering for 10 to 15 minutes or until the sauce slightly thickens.
7. Dish the curry into serving bowls and serve immediately.

TIPS:
Storage: Keep extra curry in a Tupperware and refrigerate for up to a week.
Reheat: Warm the curry in the microwave.
Serve it with: Enjoy with coconut cauliflower rice. See recipe under "Sides" segment.

NUTRITIONAL FACTS PER SERVING:
Calories: 1152 | Total Fat: 103.62g | Carbs: 8.94g | Fiber: 3.5g | Protein 48.36g

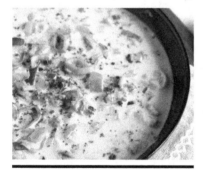

German Chicken and Cheese Soup

Macros: Fat 80% | Protein 17% | Carbs 3%
Prep time: 10 minutes | Cook time: 21 minutes | Serves: 4

This cheesy chicken soup is perfect for cold nights. Grab a bowl and watch a nice series behind the fireplace.

1 tbsp olive oil
½ lb (¼ kg) ground chicken
Salt and black pepper to taste
2 celery stalks, chopped
1 medium white onion, chopped
4 cups (946 ml) chicken stock
2/3 cup (76 g) grated Gruyere cheese
9 1/3 oz (264 g) crème fraiche
1 tsp nutmeg powder
1 tbsp fresh lemon zest

1. Heat the olive oil in a pot over medium heat and cook the chicken for 10 minutes or until no longer pink. Season with salt and black pepper.
2. Stir in the celery, onion and cook for 3 minutes or until softened.
3. Mix in the chicken stock, bring to a boil and then simmer for 8 minutes.
4. Add the cheese, crème fraiche, and nutmeg powder. Stir until the cheese melts. Adjust the taste with salt and black pepper.
5. Dish the soup into serving bowls, garnish with the lemon zest and serve warm.

TIPS:
Storage: Preserve leftover soup in a bowl, covered, and chilled for up to 2 days.
Reheat: Warm the soup in the microwave before serving.
Serve it with: Enjoy the soup with low-carb fresh bread or toasts.

NUTRITIONAL FACTS PER SERVING:
Calories: 440 | Total Fat: 39.81g | Carbs: 3.75g | Fiber: 0.5g | Protein 18.07g

Baked Beef Zoodles

Macros: Fat 70% | Protein 25% | Carbs 5%
Prep time: 15 minutes | Cook time: 30 minutes | Serves: 4

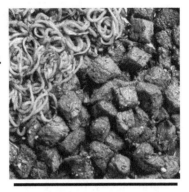

Like a one-dish pasta bake, zoodles compliments the beef mix well. It bakes quickly and is delicious.

3 tbsp olive oil
¼ lb (113 g) ground beef
Salt and black pepper to taste
½ medium onion, chopped
6 cremini mushrooms, chopped
1 garlic clove, minced
5 oz (300 ml) unsweetened tomato sauce

1 tsp dried basil
1 tsp dried oregano
2 cups (454 g) grated Monterey Jack cheese
1 cup (227 g) zoodles, spiralized zucchinis
1 tbsp chopped fresh basil to garnish

1. Heat the olive oil in a skillet over medium heat. Add the beef and cook for 10 minutes or until brown. Season with salt and black pepper.
2. Stir in the onion, mushrooms, garlic, and cook for 3 minutes or until softened.
3. Mix in the tomato sauce, basil, and oregano. Bring to a boil and then simmer for 10 minutes.
4. Meanwhile, preheat the oven to 320°F/160°C.
5. When the sauce is ready, turn the heat off and stir in the zoodles. Spoon the food into a baking dish and spread the Monterey Jack cheese on top. Bake in the oven for 7 minutes or until the cheese melts and is golden brown on top.
6. Take the dish out after, garnish with the fresh basil and serve warm.

TIPS:
Storage: Put leftovers in a Tupperware and refrigerate for up to 2 days.
Reheat: Warm food in the microwave.
Serve it with: For a light dinner, enjoy the food with low-carb cranberry juice.

NUTRITIONAL FACTS PER SERVING:
Calories: 422 | Total Fat: 33.56g | Carbs: 5.75g | Fiber: 1.5g | Protein 25.34g

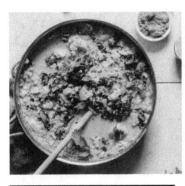

One-Pot Caulito

Macros: Fat 77% | Protein 16% | Carbs 7%
Prep time: 15 minutes | Cook time: 16 minutes | Serves: 4

Because we can't have risotto, we make caulito. This version is the fastest of a risotto style that I have made and I love that this version smells and tastes better than risotto.

2 tbsp almond oil
½ small yellow onion, chopped
2 garlic cloves, minced
1 small tomato, chopped
¼ cup vegetable broth
Salt and black pepper to taste

1 cup (227 g) cauliflower rice
1 ½ cup (340 g) grated cheddar cheese + extra for topping
2 tbsp chopped toasted almonds
1 tbsp chopped fresh parsley

TIPS:
Storage: Chill leftovers in a Tupperware for up to 2 days.
Reheat: Warm caulito in the microwave.
Serve it with: Compliment caulito with buttered mushrooms, grilled pork, or baked chicken.

NUTRITIONAL FACTS PER SERVING:
Calories: 99 | Total Fat: 5.22g | carbs: 3.48g | fiber: 1.4g | protein 5.28g

1. Heat the almond oil in a pot over medium heat.
2. Add the onion and cook for 3 minutes or until softened. Stir in the garlic and cook for 30 seconds or until fragrant.
3. Mix in the tomato, add the vegetable broth, salt, and black pepper. Bring to a boil and simmer for 5 minutes.
4. Stir in the cauliflower rice and cook covered for 5 to 7 minutes or until the liquid evaporates.
5. Pour in the cheddar cheese and stir fast until the cheese melts and the food a little sticky.
6. Dish the food, garnish with some cheddar cheese, parsley and serve warm.

Sweet Rutabaga Curry Soup

Macros: Fat 87% | Protein 9% | Carbs 4%
Prep time: 15 minutes | Cook time: 19 minutes | Serves: 4

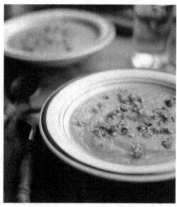

Have you heard of rutabaga before? It is a low-carb alternative to potatoes, which I love to explore in many ways. In this meal, torn between a one-bowl dish and soup, rutabagas add a lot of texture to the coconut-y base.

2 tbsp almond oil
2 tbsp butter
2 garlic cloves, minced
¼ rutabaga, peeled and chopped
1 ½ cups (355 g) coconut milk
1 ½ cups (355 g) vegetable broth
1 tbsp red curry paste

Salt and black pepper to taste
Xylitol to taste
1 cup (227 g) baby spinach
1 cup (227 g) grated cheddar cheese (white and sharp)
1 tbsp chopped fresh cilantro to garnish

1. Heat the almond oil and butter in a pot and sauté the garlic until fragrant, 30 seconds.
2. Mix in the rutabaga, coconut milk, vegetable broth, red curry paste, salt, black pepper, and xylitol. Cover, bring to a boil, and then simmer for 10 to 15 minutes or until the rutabagas are tender.
3. Open the pot and use an immersion blender to puree the soup until smooth.
4. Stir in the spinach, simmer for 2 to 3 minutes or until the spinach wilts. Adjust the taste with salt and black pepper.
5. Dish the soup into serving bowls, top with the cheddar cheese, garnish with cilantro and enjoy warm.

TIPS:
Storage: Chill soup in a Tupperware for up to 2 days.
Reheat: Warm soup in microwave, top with more cheese and enjoy!
Serve it with: Pair soup with low-carb bread for a more filling serve.

NUTRITIONAL FACTS PER SERVING:
Calories: 413 | Total Fat: 40.45g | Carbs: 4.56g | Fiber: 0.8g | Protein 9.49g

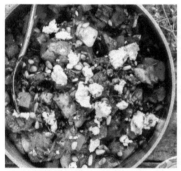

Low-Carb Ratatouille with Goat Cheese

Macros: Fat 84% | Protein 11% | Carbs 5%
Prep time: 15 minutes | Cook time: 60 minutes | Serves: 4

Some low-carb recipes may allow eggplants in ratatouille but to make this French classic shine the keto way, take out the eggplants. I incorporate as many low-carb vegetables as fit for the dish and below is the awesomeness that turned out.

2 zucchinis, diced
1 small yellow onion, chopped
1 small red bell pepper, deseeded and diced
3 garlic cloves, minced
1 tbsp fresh thyme leaves

1 tbsp fresh rosemary leaves
2 tbsp white wine vinegar
5 tbsp avocado oil
Salt and black pepper to taste
5 oz can crushed tomatoes
1 cup crumbled goat cheese

1. Preheat the oven to 400°F/200°C.
2. In a baking dish, add the zucchinis, onion, bell peppers, garlic, thyme, rosemary, vinegar, avocado oil, salt, and black pepper. Mix well and pour on the tomatoes. Stir again.
3. Bake in the oven for 45 to 60 minutes. After 30 minutes of baking, take out the dish and scatter the goat cheese on top. Continue baking to the end of the time or until the vegetables cook through.
4. Take out the dish and serve the ratatouille warm.

TIPS:
Storage: Preserve leftovers in a Tupperware and refrigerate for up to 3 days.
Reheat: Warm the ratatouille in the microwave.
Serve it with: Enjoy better with low-carb garlic bread.

NUTRITIONAL FACTS PER SERVING:
Calories: 307 | Total Fat: 28.85g | Carbs: 4.18g | Fiber: 1.3g | Protein 8.75g

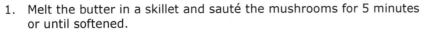

Chapter 10:Side Dishes

Garlic Cheddar Mushrooms

Macros: Fat 82% | Protein 15% | Carbs 3%
Prep time: 10 minutes | Cook time: 6 minutes | Serves: 4

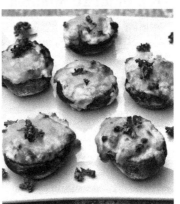

Toss some mushrooms in garlic butter, top with cheddar cheese and earn yourself a terrific side dish worthy of devouring.

3 tbsp butter
3 garlic cloves, minced
1 cup sliced cremini mushrooms
Salt and black pepper to taste

1 cup grated cheddar cheese
1 tbsp chopped fresh parsley to garnish

1. Melt the butter in a skillet and sauté the mushrooms for 5 minutes or until softened.
2. Stir in the garlic and cook for 30 seconds or until fragrant.
3. Dish the food onto serving plates, top with the Parmesan cheese and garnish with the parsley. Serve warm.

NUTRITIONAL FACTS PER SERVING:
Calories: 199 | Total Fat: 18.27g | Carbs: 1.76g | Fiber: 0.3g | Protein 7.59g

TIPS:
Storage: Keep leftovers in a Tupperware and refrigerate for up to 4 days.
Reheat: Warm in the microwave.
Serve it with: Add a kick to the mushrooms with some red chili flakes. Serve as a side to meat dishes.

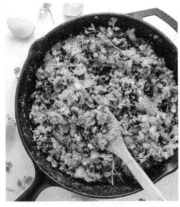

Mexican Cauli-Rice

Macros: Fat 82% | Protein 13% | Carbs 5%
Prep time: 10 minutes | Cook time: 6 minutes | Serves: 4

You can alternate between cauli fried rice and Mexican friend rice for your stew dishes.

2 tbsp butter
2 tbsp almond oil
½ tsp onion flakes
3 garlic cloves, minced
1 tbsp unsweetened tomato puree

1 cup (227 g) cauliflower rice
Salt and black pepper to taste
1 cup grated Mexican cheese blend
2 tbsp chopped fresh cilantro

TIPS:
Storage: Keep leftovers in a Tupperware and refrigerate for up to a week.
Reheat: Warm in the microwave.
Serve it with: Serve as a side to stews and meat dishes.

1. Heat the butter and almond oil in a pot and sauté the onion flakes and garlic for 30 seconds or until fragrant.
2. Mix in the tomato puree and cook for 2 minutes.
3. Stir in the cauliflower rice, add a quarter cup of water, salt, black pepper, and simmer for 3 to 4 minutes or until the cauliflower softens.
4. Stir in the Mexican cheese blend afterwards and dish the food. Garnish with the cilantro and serve warm.

NUTRITIONAL FACTS PER SERVING:
Calories: 223 | Total Fat: 20.64g | Carbs: 3.04g | Fiber: 0.7g | Protein 7.39g

Garlic Sautéed Rapini

Macros: Fat 83% | Protein 14% | Carbs 3%
Prep time: 10 minutes | Cook time: 11 minutes | Serves: 4

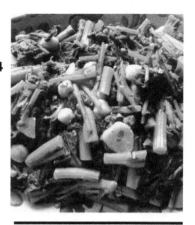

We love greens, don't we? Sauté some rapini, mustard leaves, spinach, kale, or whichever you like with garlic and serve it as a side to many main dishes.

2 tbsp avocado oil
4 garlic cloves, minced
2 cups (454 g) rapini
Salt to taste

1 cup (227 g) grated Monterey Jack cheese for topping
2 tbsp toasted almond flakes for topping

1. Heat the avocado oil in a large skillet and sauté the garlic until fragrant, 30 seconds.
2. Mix in the rapini and cook for 8 to 10 minutes or until tender. Season with salt.
3. Dish the rapini onto serving plates, top with the Monterey Jack cheese, almonds, and serve immediately.

NUTRITIONAL FACTS PER SERVING:
Calories: 254 | Total Fat: 23.91g | Carbs: 1.79g | Fiber: 0.6g | Protein 8.9g

TIPS:
Storage: Keep leftovers in a Tupperware and refrigerate for up to a week.
Reheat: Warm in the microwave.
Serve it with: Add the rapini as a compliment to several meat dishes.

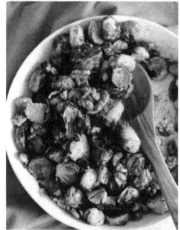

Crispy Roasted Brussels Sprouts and Walnuts

Macros: Fat 95% | Protein 1% | Carbs 4%
Prep time: 15 minutes | Cook time: 14 minutes | Serves: 4

Brussels sprouts are low in carbs and we love them! This walnut-combo sauté is an exciting way to enjoy them.

3 tbsp almond oil
1/3 lb (151.3 g) Brussels sprouts, halved
2 garlic cloves, minced
1 red chili pepper, deseeded and minced
2 sprigs chopped fresh mint

¼ cup (59 ml) coconut aminos
1 tbsp xylitol
1 tbsp plain vinegar
1 tbsp toasted sesame seeds
½ cup (113 g) chopped toasted walnuts
Salt to taste

TIPS:
Storage: Keep leftovers in a Tupperware and refrigerate for up to 5 days.
Reheat: Warm in the microwave.
Serve it with: Serve the vegetables with grilled, baked, or braised meats.

1. Heat the sesame oil in a large skillet and sauté the Brussels sprouts for 10 minutes or until softened.
2. Stir in the garlic, red chili pepper, and mint leaves for 1 minute or until fragrant.
3. In a bowl, mix the coconut aminos, xylitol, and vinegar. Pour the mixture over the vegetables and toss well. Simmer for 1 to 2 minutes.
4. Mix in the sesame seeds, walnuts, and adjust the taste with salt as needed.
5. Dish the food onto serving plates and enjoy!

NUTRITIONAL FACTS PER SERVING:
Calories: 351 | Total Fat: 37.73g | Carbs: 3.93g | Fiber: 1.5g | Protein 1.42g

Spicy Butter Baked Asparagus

Macros: Fat 83% | Protein 13% | Carbs 4%
Prep time: 15 minutes | Cook time: 15 minutes | Serves: 4

An alternate way to preparing asparagus to have an excellent flavor.

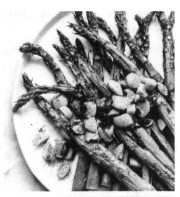

½ lb (227 g) asparagus, hard stems removed
½ cup (113 g) salted butter, melted

1 tsp cayenne pepper
Salt and black pepper to taste
1 cup grated Monterey Jack cheese for topping

1. Preheat the oven to 425°F/220°C.
2. Spread the asparagus on a baking tray.
3. In a small bowl, mix the butter, cayenne pepper, salt, and black pepper. Drizzle the mixture on the asparagus and toss well with a spatula. Scatter the Monterey Jack cheese on top.
4. Bake in the oven for 15 minutes or until golden brown and the asparagus are tender. Serve afterwards.

NUTRITIONAL FACTS PER SERVING:
Calories: 253 | Total Fat: 24.01g | Carbs: 2.66g | Fiber: 1.3g | Protein 8.38g

TIPS:
Storage: Keep leftovers in a bowl and refrigerate for up to a week.
Reheat: Warm in the microwave.
Serve it with: The asparagus serve best with grilled, baked, or braised meats.

Wild Garlic Skillet Bread

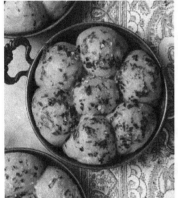

Macros: Fat 97% | Protein 0% | Carbs 2%
Prep time: 1 hour 50 minutes | Cook time: 25 minutes | Serves: 4

Many of the soup recipes in this cookbook call for enjoying the soup with low-carb bread. Here is one fantastic option to indulge.

3 ¼ cups almond flour + extra for dusting
¼ tsp erythritol
¾ tsp salt
¾ oz agar agar powder

1 cup lukewarm water
3/8 cup melted butter + extra for greasing
1 cup chopped fresh wild garlic
Flaky salt for topping

TIPS:
Storage: Place leftover bread in a plastic bag and freeze for up to a week.
Reheat: Warm bread in a preheated oven or microwave.
Serve it with: Enjoy the bread with stews and soups.

NUTRITIONAL FACTS PER SERVING:
Calories: 1893 | Total Fat: 208.42g | Carbs: 11.61g | Fiber: 0.7g | Protein 2.37g

1. In a mixer's bowl, using the dough hook, mix the almond flour, erythritol, salt, and agar agar powder. Add the lukewarm water and combine until dough forms.
2. Dust a surface with almond flour, add the dough and knead with your hands until smooth and elastic.
3. Brush a bowl with melted butter, sit in the dough and cover with a damp napkin. Put the bowl on top of your refrigerator and let rise for 1 hour.
4. After, take off the napkin and press the dough with your fist to release the air trapped in the dough. Divide the dough into 12 pieces and re-shape into a ball.
5. Grease an oven-proof skillet with olive oil and arrange the dough rolls in the pan. Cover with a damp napkin and let rise again for 30 minutes.
6. Take off the napkin, brush the top of the dough with olive oil, and sprinkle with the wild garlic leaves and some flaky salt.
7. Preheat the oven to 400°F/200°C.
8. Place the skillet in the oven and bake for 20 to 25 minutes or until golden brown.
9. Remove the skillet, let cool and then enjoy the bread!

Grilled Zucchini with Pecan Gremolata

Macros: Fat 89% | Protein 10% | Carbs 1%
Prep time: 45 minutes | Cook time: 8 minutes | Serves: 4

A side dish that can serve as a main because it is quickly filling. It is an excellent option for vegan and vegetarian keto dieting.

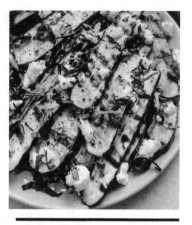

2 zucchinis, cut into strips
Salt and black pepper to taste
4 tbsp sugar-free maple syrup
½ cup (113 g) olive oil, divided
2 scallions, chopped
8 garlic cloves, minced

1 cup (227 g) toasted pecans, chopped
8 tbsp pork rinds
2 tbsp chopped fresh parsley
1 tbsp plain vinegar

1. Sprinkle the zucchinis with salt and let sit for 15 to 30 minutes to release liquid. After, pat dry with a paper towel. In a bowl, mix 2 tablespoons of olive oil with the maple syrup and toss with the zucchinis.
2. Heat a grill pan over medium heat and grill the zucchinis on both sides for 3 to 4 minutes per side or until golden brown. Remove onto a serving platter.
3. In a bowl, mix the remaining olive oil, scallions, garlic, pecans, pork rinds, parsley, and vinegar. Spoon the gremolata all over the zucchinis and enjoy!

NUTRITIONAL FACTS PER SERVING:
Calories: 1852 | Total Fat: 184.1g | Carbs: 5.7g | Fiber: 1.4g | Protein 43.88g

TIPS:
Storage: Separately keep leftover zucchinis and gremolata in bowls and refrigerate for up to 5 days.
Reheat: Heat zucchinis in the microwave and warm gremolata at room temperature.
Serve it with: Pair the zucchinis and gremolata with grilled steak, pork chops, or chicken.

Coconut Cauli Fried Rice

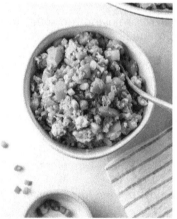

Macros: Fat 73% | Protein 21% | Carbs 5%
Prep time: 10 minutes | Cook time: 8 minutes | Serves: 4

Cauli fried rice is an essential side dish on the keto diet. It pairs well with many meat and stew dishes. Therefore, I made sure to load it well with enough vegetables and seasoning.

2 tbsp coconut oil
1 small red bell pepper, deseeded and chopped
1 scallion, chopped + extra for garnish
2 garlic cloves, minced

4 eggs, beaten
1 cup (227 g) cauliflower rice
1 tbsp coconut aminos
Salt and black pepper to taste
1 cup grated cheddar cheese

TIPS:
Storage: Put leftovers in a bowl and refrigerate for up to 5 days.
Reheat: Warm in a microwave.
Serve it with: Add the cauliflower fried rice as a compliment to meats and sauce dishes.

1. Melt the coconut oil in wok and stir-fry the bell peppers for 5 minutes or tender.
2. Mix in the scallions, garlic and cook for 30 seconds or until fragrant.
3. Add the eggs to the wok and scramble until set. Mix in the cauliflower rice and cook for 1 to 2 minutes or until the cauliflower rice is tender with a bite to the teeth.
4. Stir in the coconut aminos, sesame seeds, and adjust the taste with salt and black pepper. Simmer for 1 minute and stir in the cheddar cheese. Turn the heat off and serve immediately.

NUTRITIONAL FACTS PER SERVING:
Calories: 251 | Total Fat: 20.68g | Carbs: 3.63g | Fiber: 1g | Protein 13.11g

Mini Parsnip Pancakes

Macros: Fat 90% | Protein 5% | Carbs 4%
Prep time: 15 minutes | Cook time: 24 minutes | Serves: 4

Bring breakfast to dinner and enjoy these pancakes with many stew dishes.

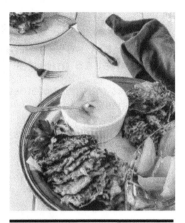

1 parsnip, finely grated
1 small white onions, finely grated
¼ tsp nutmeg powder
Salt and black pepper to taste
2 eggs

1 cup (227 g) almond flour
1 cup (227 g) grated cheddar cheese
4 tbsp avocado oil for frying

1. In a bowl, mix the parsnip, onions, nutmeg powder, salt, black pepper, eggs, almond flour, and Monterey Jack cheese until well-combined.
2. Heat the avocado oil in a large skillet over medium heat.
3. Working in batches, use a scoop to add drops of the mixture into the skillet with intervals. Press down to form patties and fry on both sides for 3 to 4 minutes per side or until golden brown and compacted.
4. Remove the pancakes to a paper towel-lined plate to drain grease and make more pancakes.

TIPS:
Storage: Preserve leftover pancakes in a bowl and chill for up to 4 days.
Reheat: Warm in the microwave.
Serve it with: Enjoy the pancakes with sauces, stews, and meat dishes.

NUTRITIONAL FACTS PER SERVING:
Calories: 784 | Total Fat: 79.88g | Carbs: 8.97g | Fiber: 1.7g | Protein 10.28g

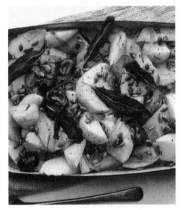

Korean Braised Turnips

Macros: Fat 75% | Protein 19% | Carbs 5%
Prep time: 15 minutes | Cook time: 27 minutes | Serves: 4

Braise some turnips with coconut aminos and peanut oil to experience the Korean lifestyle right in your home.

1 large turnip, peeled and cubed
2 tbsp almond oil
2 garlic cloves, minced
6 tbsp coconut aminos

3 tbsp swerve brown sugar
½ cup (125 ml) vegetable broth
1 cup grated Gruyere cheese

1. Add the turnip to a pot and cover with slightly salted water. Boil over medium heat for 5 minutes or slightly tender. Drain the turnips.
2. Heat the almond oil in a deep skillet and sauté the garlic until fragrant, 30 seconds.
3. In a bowl, mix the coconut aminos and swerve brown sugar.
4. Toss the turnips in the peanut oil and pour on the coconut aminos mixture. Sauté for 1 minute and add the vegetable broth. Stir well and cook for 20 minutes or until the turnips soften and the liquid reduces.
5. Spoon the turnips onto serving plates, top with the Gruyere cheese and garnish with the peanuts.

TIPS:
Storage: Keep leftovers in a Tupperware and refrigerate for up to a week.
Reheat: Warm in the microwave.
Serve it with: Enjoy the turnips with a wide range of meat dishes and sauces.

NUTRITIONAL FACTS PER SERVING:
Calories: 182 | Total Fat: 15.57g | Carbs: 2.55g | Fiber: 0.6g | Protein 8.42g

Creamy Mashed Cauliflower

Macros: Fat 96% | Protein 1% | Carbs 3%
Prep time: 15 minutes | Cook time: 12 minutes | Serves: 4

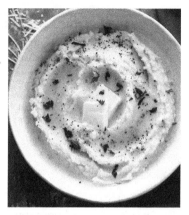

It replaces mashed potatoes as a requisite side dish for many meat and stew dishes.

2 (236 g) head cauliflowers, cut into florets
1 cup (227 g) almond milk
1/3 cup (74 g) heavy cream
4 garlic cloves, minced
¼ tsp nutmeg powder

Salt and black pepper to taste
4 tbsp unsalted butter, room temperature
2 tbsp cream cheese
1 tbsp chopped fresh scallions

1. Add the cauliflower and about 2 cups of salted water to a pot, cover, and bring to a boil over medium heat. Reduce the heat and simmer for 10 minutes or until the cauliflower is tender. Drain the cauliflower and pour into a bowl.
2. Meanwhile as the cauliflower cooked, pour the almond milk in a pot and add the heavy cream, garlic, nutmeg powder, salt, and black pepper. Warm over medium-low heat for 1 to 2 minutes but don't let boil.
3. Mash the cauliflower using a masher until smooth. Add the butter, cream cheese, and pour the warm almond milk mixture. Mix well until the butter and cream cheese melt and combine well with the other ingredients.
4. Garnish with the scallions and serve warm.

TIPS:
Storage: Put leftovers in a Tupperware and refrigerate for up to 5 days.
Reheat: Warm mashed cauliflower in the microwave.
Serve it with: You may swap cauliflower for turnips, rutabagas, parsnips, celeriac, or broccoli. Serve the mashed cauliflower with a variety of meat and sauce mains.

NUTRITIONAL FACTS PER SERVING:
Calories: 662 | Total Fat: 72.08g | Carbs: 5.02g | Fiber: 1.5g | Protein 2.36g

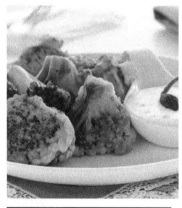

Broccoli Fried Cheese

Macros: Fat 77% | Protein 22% | Carbs 1%
Prep time: 15 minutes | Cook time: 14 minutes | Serves: 4

I love having this food with fried chicken to replace French fries but I find myself snacking on them sometimes.

1 (225 g) head broccoli, cut into florets
2 eggs
1 cup (227 g) grated cheddar cheese

1/3 cup (74 g) grated Monterey Jack cheese
2 tbsp butter

TIPS:
Storage: Keep leftovers in a bowl and refrigerate for up to a week.
Reheat: Warm in the microwave.
Serve it with: Enjoy with many meat and sauce dishes as a side.

1. Add the broccoli to a steamer and cook for 10 minutes or until tender.
2. Pour the broccoli into a bowl and let cool. Crack on the eggs and mix with the cheeses.
3. Working the batches, melt the butter in a large skillet and fry the broccoli on both sides for 3 to 4 minutes per side or until golden brown.
4. Remove the broccoli to a plate and serve warm.

NUTRITIONAL FACTS PER SERVING:
Calories: 240 | Total Fat: 20.75g | Carbs: 0.9g | Fiber: 0.3g | Protein 12.6g

Bell Pepper Rings with Cheddar Dipping Sauce

Macros: Fat 86% | Protein 13% | Carbs 1%
Prep time: 20 minutes | Cook time: 26 minutes | Serves: 4

We've had onion rings for days, at the restaurants, snack bags, friend's parties, and so on. Here's time for a change and luckily, these bell pepper version tastes better and smells sweeter. To lift up the fatty counts, the pairing cheddar dipping sauce is one not to ignore.

Bell Pepper Rings:
1 large red bell pepper
½ cup (113 g) almond flour
2 eggs, beaten
2 cups (454 g) crushed pork rinds

1 tsp salt
2 tsp paprika
½ tsp allspice powder
½ tsp ginger powder

Cheddar Dipping Sauce:
2 tbsp butter
1 tbsp almond flour
1 cup (227 g) almond milk
2 tbsp heavy cream

1 tsp salt
1 cup (227 g) grated cheddar cheese (white and sharp)
1 tsp prepared mustard

Bell pepper rings:
1. Preheat the oven to 350°F/180°C and line a baking tray with greaseproof paper.
2. Cut off the heads of the bell pepper and use a small knife to score out the seeds and membrane. After, slice the peppers into rings.
3. Pour the almond flour on a plate and beat the eggs in a wide bowl. Add the pork rinds to a plate and mix with the salt, paprika, allspice powder, and ginger powder.
4. Dust the peppers in the almond flour, dip in the egg, and then generously coat in the pork rinds.
5. Arrange the pepper rings on the baking tray and bake in the oven for 15 to 20 minutes or until the peppers are golden brown and crispy.
6. Meanwhile, make the dipping sauce.

Cheddar dipping sauce:
1. Melt the butter in a medium pot over medium heat and whisk in the almond flour.
2. Pour in the almond milk and mix until smooth. Stir in the heavy cream, salt, cheddar cheese, and mustard until the cheese melts. Turn the heat off.
3. Pour the dipping sauce into serving bowls and serve with the bell pepper rings when ready.

TIPS:
Storage: Keep bell pepper rings in a plastic zipper bag and refrigerate for up to 3 days. Chill sauce in the fridge too.
Reheat: Warm pepper rings in preheated oven for 3 to 5 minutes and serve with chilled dipping sauce.
Serve it with: For a fuller platter, add some onion rings, mozzarella sticks, and celery sticks while serving.

NUTRITIONAL FACTS PER SERVING:
Calories: 1690 | Total Fat: 161.48g | Carbs: 3.36g | Fiber: 0.7g | Protein 54.2g

Crispy Chicken Skin with Parmesan Dipping Sauce

Macros: Fat 88% | Protein 11% | Carbs 1%
Prep time: 15 minutes | Cook time: 20 minutes | Serves: 4

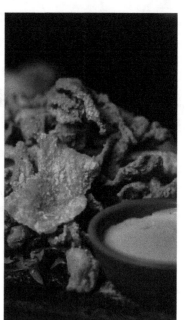

Now, you can gather all those chicken breasts skins that you would have removed and discarded. You see, beneath and within chicken skin sits a good amount of healthy fats, which is essential for the keto diet. These crispy crackles are an excellent way to reap all the nutrients of your chicken.

Crispy Chicken:
1 tsp erythritol
5 tbsp plain vinegar
5 tsp coconut aminos
2 tbsp unsweetened tomato sauce
1 tsp salt

1 tbsp onion powder
1 garlic clove, pressed
1 lb (454g) chicken skin
Olive oil for frying

Parmesan Dipping Sauce:
½ cup mayonnaise
1 tsp olive oil
1 ½ tsp swerve sugar
2 tbsp plain vinegar

2 garlic cloves, crushed
2 tbsp grated Parmesan cheese
¼ tsp dried basil
Salt and black pepper to taste

Crispy chicken:
1. In a medium bowl, mix the erythritol, vinegar, coconut aminos, tomato sauce, salt, onion powder, and garlic. Add the chicken skin and toss well until thoroughly coated. Marinate in the refrigerator for at least 1 hour.
2. Afterwards, heat some olive oil in a deep pan. Working in batches, fry the chicken skin for 5 to 10 minutes or until golden brown and crispy, turning halfway. Remove the chicken onto a paper towel-lined plate to drain grease and set aside to cool while you prepare the dipping sauce.

Parmesan dipping sauce:
1. In a bowl, mix the mayonnaise, olive oil, swerve sugar, vinegar, garlic, Parmesan cheese, basil, salt, and black pepper.
2. Serve the crispy chicken with the dipping sauce.

TIPS:
Storage: Preserve crispy chicken in a plastic zipper bag and refrigerate for up to a week.
Reheat: Warm chicken in the microwave or deep-fry for 2 to 3 minutes to maintain crunch.
Serve it with: Enjoy better with French fries or celery sticks.

NUTRITIONAL FACTS PER SERVING:
Calories: 609 | Total Fat: 59.13g | Carbs: 1.68g | Fiber: 0.2g | Protein 16.34g

Cheesy Zucchini Triangles with Garlic Mayo Dip

Macros: Fat 91% | Protein 4% | Carbs 5%
Prep time: 20 minutes | Cook time: 30 minutes | Serves: 4

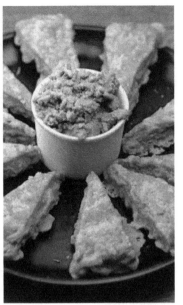

Sometimes upping your game on regular zucchini sticks could give you a win at the table. The inspiration for these triangles come from traditional zucchini sticks but made into a pizza. The crust is thin and crunchy. Enjoying them as they are is tasty but paired with this garlic mayo dip is mind-blowing.

Garlic Mayo Dip:
1 cup (227 g) crème fraiche
1/3 cup (80 g) mayonnaise
¼ tsp sugar-free maple syrup
1 garlic clove, pressed
½ tsp vinegar
Salt and black pepper to taste

Cheesy Zucchini Triangles:
2 large zucchinis, grated
1 egg
¼ cup (20 g) almond flour
¼ tsp paprika powder
¾ tsp dried mixed herbs
¼ tsp swerve sugar
½ cup (113.5 g) grated mozzarella cheese

1. Start by making the dip; in a medium bowl, mix the crème fraiche, mayonnaise, maple syrup, garlic, vinegar, salt, and black pepper. Cover the bowl with a plastic wrap and refrigerate while you make the zucchinis.
2. Preheat the oven to 400°F/200°C and line a baking tray with greaseproof paper. Set aside.
3. Put the zucchinis in a cheesecloth and press out as much liquid as possible. Pour the zucchinis in a bowl.
4. Add the egg, almond flour, paprika, dried mixed herbs, and swerve sugar. Mix well and spread the mixture on the baking tray into a round pizza-like piece with 1-inch thickness. Bake in the oven for 25 minutes or until golden brown and crispy.
5. Reduce the oven's heat to 350°F/175°C, take out the tray and sprinkle the zucchini with the mozzarella cheese. Return the tray to the oven and bake for 5 minutes or until the cheese melts.
6. Remove afterwards, set aside to cool for 5 minutes and then slice the snacks into triangles. Serve immediately with the garlic mayo dip.

TIPS:
Storage: Keep extra zucchini triangles in a plastic zipper bag and refrigerate for up to a week. Preserve the dip in the refrigerator.
Reheat: Warm the zucchini triangles in the microwave and serve with the chilled dip.
Serve it with: You can also enjoy the zucchini triangles with a three-cheese dip.

NUTRITIONAL FACTS PER SERVING:
Calories: 401 | Total Fat: 41.14g | Carbs: 4.94g | Fiber: 0.2g | Protein 4.08g

Turnip Latkes with Creamy Avocado Sauce

Macros: Fat 88% | Protein 7% | Carbs 5%
Prep time: 20 minutes | Cook time: 16 minutes | Serves: 4

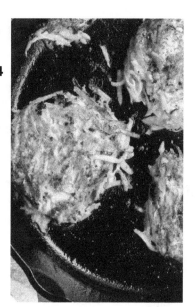

A crunchy, filling piece is essential for keto snacking. These cheese-infused latkes paired with a tasty dip are excellent for mid-day or late night snacking. They are crispy on the outside and chewy on the inside for the right treat.

Turnip Latkes:
½ lb (227 g) turnips, peeled and shredded
1 tbsp almond flour
1 shallot, minced
1 egg

½ cup (113 g) grated cheddar cheese (white and sharp)
Salt and black pepper to taste
5 tbsp almond oil for frying

Creamy Avocado Sauce:
½ avocado, pitted and peeled
1 ½ up (340.5 g) Greek yogurt
½ tsp vinegar
1 small garlic clove, minced

1 tbsp avocado oil
1 tbsp chopped fresh cilantro
Salt and black pepper to taste

Turnip Latkes:
1. Place the turnips in a cheesecloth, fold up and press out as much liquid as possible.
2. Pour the turnips into a bowl and add the almond flour, shallot, egg, cheddar cheese, salt, and black pepper. Mix well and form 1-inch patties from the mixture.
3. Heat the almond oil in a non-stick skillet over medium heat. Working in batches, add 4 to 6 patties and cook for 4 to 5 minutes or until golden brown beneath. Turn the latkes and cook the other side for 3 to 4 minutes or until golden brown too.
4. Remove the latkes onto a paper towel-lined plate to drain grease and fry the remaining patties.

Dill Yogurt Sauce:
1. Mash the avocado in a medium bowl. Mix in the Greek yogurt, vinegar, garlic, avocado oil, cilantro, salt, and black pepper.
2. Serve the latkes with the avocado sauce.

TIPS:
Storage: Preserve extra latkes in a Tupperware and refrigerate for up to a week. Also, cover avocado sauce with plastic wrap and refrigerate for the same period.
Reheat: Warm latkes in the microwave and serve with the chilled avocado sauce.
Serve it with: You can have a medley of sauces of the latkes like dill yogurt sauce and spicy mayo.

NUTRITIONAL FACTS PER SERVING:
Calories: 518 | Total Fat: 51.78g | Carbs: 6.96g | Fiber: 3.6g | Protein 8.78g

Nutty Bars

Macros: Fat 90% | Protein 4% | Carbs 5%
Prep time: 10 minutes | Cook time: 20 minutes | Serves: 4

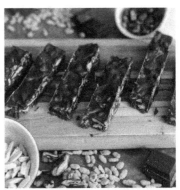

Are nutty bars overrated? I don't think so. Nothing screams keto better than a blend of many keto-certified nuts, made into crunchy bars to be enjoyed for days. Mind you, these pieces contain some coconut flakes and peanut butter to make things all the better.

2/3 cup almond flour
¼ tsp salt
2 cups mixed toasted nuts
¼ cup unsweetened coconut flakes

½ tbsp chia seeds
2 tbsp creamy peanut butter
2 tbsp almond oil
1/3 cup sugar-free maple syrup

TIPS:
Storage: Keep extra nutty bars in an airtight jar (covered) at room temperature for up to a week.
Reheat: None required.
Serve it with: Crunch on them as they are.

1. Preheat the oven to 300°F/150°C and line a baking tray with greaseproof paper. Set aside.
2. In a medium bowl, mix the almond flour, salt, nuts, coconut flakes, and chia seeds. Add the peanut butter, almond oil, maple syrup, and mix well.
3. Spread the mixture on the baking tray into a 1 ½-inch thick rectangle. Bake in the oven for 20 minutes or until the bar is compact.
4. Once ready, remove from the oven, slightly cool and enjoy the bars.

NUTRITIONAL FACTS PER SERVING:
Calories: 911 | Total Fat: 95.69g | Carbs: 12.08g | Fiber: 4.1g | Protein 11.62g

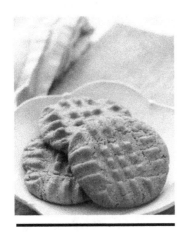

Easy Peanut Butter Cookies

Macros: Fat 91% | Protein 5% | Carbs 4%
Prep time: 15 minutes | Cook time: 10 minutes | Serves: 4

Making cookies shouldn't be intimidating and these peanut butter ones teach us so. With only four main ingredients, a happy heart and a ready tummy to consume, you will be making such crunchy and sweet-smelling cookies.

1/3 cup (76 g) creamy peanut butter
½ cup almond flour
1 egg

3 tbsp almond oil
¾ cup (155 g) xylitol
2 pinches of salt

TIPS:
Storage: Preserve extra cookies in an airtight jar and keep for up to a week.
Reheat: None required.
Serve it with: Enjoy with a warm or cold glass of almond milk.

1. Preheat the oven to 350°F/180°C and line a baking tray with greaseproof paper.
2. In a bowl, mix the peanut butter, almond flour, egg, almond oil, xylitol, and salt.
3. Put 2-tablespoon mounds of the batter on the baking tray with intervals. Use a fork to slightly press down on the cookies at two 90-degree angles to create a marked design.
4. Bake in the oven for 10 minutes or until the cookies firm up. Take out of the oven and cool for 5 minutes.
5. Transfer to a wire rack to completely cool and enjoy!

NUTRITIONAL FACTS PER SERVING:
Calories: 463 | Total Fat: 48.11g | Carbs: 4.69g | Fiber: 1.4g | Protein 6.45g

Maple Candied Bacon

Macros: Fat 78% | Protein 21% | Carbs 1%
Prep time: 10 minutes | Cook time: 20 minutes | Serves: 4

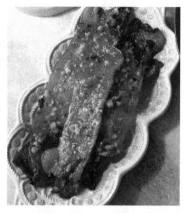

What better way to express your love than with candied bacon? It is an excellent way to share your keto journey with your non-keto family or loved ones. Sweet and savory with a bit of heat that's enjoyable as a snack or a compliment for a brunch platter.

2 tbsp melted butter
1 tbsp almond oil
¼ cup (48 ml) sugar-free maple syrup

1 tbsp (20 g) swerve brown sugar
¼ tsp cayenne pepper
Salt to taste
4 bacon slices

1. Preheat the oven to 350°F/180°C and line a baking tray with greaseproof paper. Set aside.
2. In a bowl, mix the butter, almond oil, maple syrup, swerve brown sugar, cayenne pepper, and salt. Lay the bacon on the baking tray and brush both sides with the syrup mixture.
3. Bake in the oven for 15 to 20 minutes or until the bacon is golden brown and crispy.
4. Remove from the oven afterwards, let cool and enjoy.

TIPS:
Storage: Preserve extras in a plastic zipper bag and chill for up to 5 days.
Reheat: None required
Serve it with: Crunch on them as they are.

NUTRITIONAL FACTS PER SERVING:
Calories: 113 | Total Fat: 9.97g | Carbs: 0.44g | Fiber: 0g | Protein 5.84g

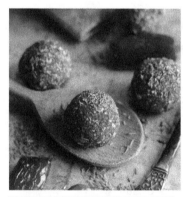

Walnut Cinnamon Balls

Macros: Fat 90% | Protein 5% | Carbs 5%
Prep time: 20 minutes | Chilling time: 1 hour | Serves: 12

They are that pampering, mind-relaxing treat at midday. These pieces boost the body with so much energy. Thanks to their chewy, crunchy feel, they make you want to have them almost always.

1 oz (28 g) goji berries or dried cranberries
2 cups (454 g) toasted walnuts
3 tbsp unsweetened coconut flakes

A pinch cinnamon powder
Salt to taste
3 tbsp almond oil

TIPS:
Storage: Preserve extra snack balls in an airtight container at room temperature for up to 5 days.
Reheat: None required.
Serve it with: Enjoy with fresh berry juice.

1. Line a cookie tray with greaseproof paper.
2. Add all the ingredients to a food processor and blend until coarsely smooth.
3. Roll bite-size balls out of the mixture and arrange on the cookie sheet with intervals. Refrigerate for at least 1 hour or until the balls are compacted.

NUTRITIONAL FACTS PER SERVING:
Calories: 444 | Total Fat: 46.51g | Carbs: 6.03g | Fiber: 2.8g | Protein 6.14g

Frozen Strawberry Yogurt Bites

Macros: Fat 92% | Protein 3% | Carbs 5%
Prep time: 10 minutes | Freezing time: 4 hours | Serves: 10

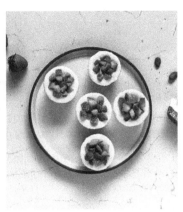

I love sucking on these as a late night snack, especially on warm nights. They are soothing, straightforward to make, and you can keep them for days.

¼ cup (75 g) fresh or frozen strawberries
2 tbsp sugar-free maple syrup, divided
½ tsp vinegar
2 cups (150 g) Greek yogurt

1. Place the strawberries, maple syrup, and vinegar in a bowl. Use an immersion blender to process the ingredients until smooth.
2. Spoon the mixture into the holes of an ice-cube tray, halfway up. Top with the Greek yogurt to the rim of the holes. Spread out to be even and freeze for at least 4 hours.
3. Enjoy the snack ice cold.

NUTRITIONAL FACTS PER SERVING:
Calories: 106 | Total Fat: 10.47g | Carbs: 3.79g | Fiber: 1g | Protein 1.23g

TIPS:
Storage: Keep remaining bites in the freezer for up to 1 month.
Reheat: None required.
Serve it with: Blend bites into a berry smoothie or use for garnishing a smoothie bowl.

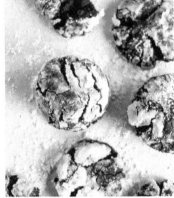

Dark Chocolate Crinkle Crackers

Macros: Fat 96% | Protein 2% | Carbs 2%
Prep time: 15 minutes | Cook time: 12 minutes | Chilling time: 1 hour | Serves: 4

I remember making these pieces for my daughter's end-of-year party at school. It felt so bad to have some of the non-keto version. And then, I realized I could make a keto-type for myself. Here are the crunchy pieces I made. Make sure to make plenty because it is quite addictive.

1 cup almond flour
¾ tsp baking powder
2 tbsp unsweetened cocoa powder
¾ tsp salt
¼ cup dark chocolate, roughly chopped
2 tbsp butter, room temperature
1 egg
½ cup swerve sugar
1 tsp vanilla extract
¼ cup swerve confectioner's sugar

TIPS:
Storage: Preserve extra cookies in an airtight jar and keep for up to a week.
Reheat: None required.
Serve it with: Enjoy with a warm or cold glass of almond milk.

NUTRITIONAL FACTS PER SERVING:
Calories: 595 | Total Fat: 64.37g | Carbs: 4.68g | Fiber: 1.7g | Protein 2.46g

1. In a medium bowl, mix the almond flour, baking powder, cocoa powder, and salt. Set aside.
2. Double-boil the chocolate until melted and mix in the butter until melted too.
3. Add the egg, swerve sugar, and vanilla to a large bowl and whisk with electric beaters until fluffy.
4. After, mix in the chocolate and dry ingredients until smooth batter forms. Cover the bowl with a plastic wrap and refrigerate for at least 2 hours.
5. Preheat the oven to 350°F/180°C and line a baking tray with greaseproof paper.
6. Take the batter out of the refrigerator and form into bite-size balls. Roll the pieces in the swerve confectioner's sugar and arrange on the baking tray.
7. Bake in the oven for 12 minutes.
8. Take out of the oven when ready, let cool and enjoy.

Blueberry Swiss Roll

Macros: Fat 90% | Protein 6% | Carbs 4%
Prep time: 15 minutes | Cook time: 10 minutes | Serves: 4

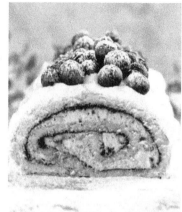

I call it a loaded omelet filled with goodness. This dessert astounds you! The fluffy base is a delight to bite into, which oozes vanilla-flavored cream and a blueberry reveal.

2 egg whites, separated
¼ cup (57 g) swerve sugar
2 egg yolks
2 tbsp water
2 tsp vanilla extract
¼ cup (57 g) almond flour
¼ cup (57 g) xanthan gum

¼ tsp baking powder
1 cup (237 ml) heavy cream
Swerve confectioner's sugar for topping
¼ cup fresh blueberries

1. Preheat the oven to 400°F/200°C.
2. Beat the egg whites in a mixer until foamy. Add half of the swerve sugar and beat until stiff peaks form.
3. In a bowl, whisk the egg yolks, remaining swerve sugar, water, and vanilla. Sieve in the almond flour, xanthan gum, baking powder, and whisk until well-incorporated. Add the egg whites mixture and combine well.
4. Line a baking sheet with greaseproof paper and spread the mixture on top. Bake in the oven for 8 to 10 minutes or until set and golden brown.
5. Sprinkle some swerve confectioner's sugar on clean napkin, remove the cake onto the napkin, and roll on top. Set aside.
6. Meanwhile, whisk the heavy cream and remaining swerve confectioner's sugar until smooth.
7. Unroll the cake, spread the heavy cream mix on top and scatter the blueberries on the cream. Slice and serve immediately.

TIPS:
Storage: Refrigerate leftovers for up to 3 days.
Reheat: None required.
Serve it with: Add some low-carb vanilla ice cream on top and enjoy!

NUTRITIONAL FACTS PER SERVING:
Calories: 271 | Total Fat: 27.04g | Carbs: 2.87g | Fiber: 0.2g | Protein 3.83g

Vanilla Pudding with Warm Strawberries

Macros: Fat 95% | Protein 2% | Carbs 3%
Prep time: 15 minutes | Cook time: 58 minutes | Serves: 4

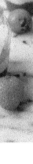

Adding warmed strawberries with sauce to what will have been a normal vanilla pudding is the exciting factor here. The pudding is smooth and creamy with chunky strawberries warmed in a red wine sauce for lots of aroma.

Vanilla pudding:
1 ¾ cups (400 ml) almond milk
1 cup (237 ml) heavy cream
¾ cup (150 g) swerve sugar
1 vanilla bean, paste extracted

A pinch of salt
1 egg
5 egg yolks

Warm strawberries:
½ cup (113 ml) red wine
1 tsp strawberry extract
1 cinnamon stick
1 tsp xanthan gum

A pinch salt
2 cups (454 g) fresh strawberries, halved

Vanilla pudding:
1. Preheat the oven to 230°F/110°C.
2. In a pot, add the almond milk, heavy cream, a third of the swerve sugar, vanilla paste, and salt. Bring the mixture to a boil over medium heat and turn the heat off.
3. Whisk the egg, egg yolks, and another third of the swerve sugar.
4. Pour the cream mixture into the eggs and vigorously whisk until well combined.
5. Divide the mixture into mini baking cups and bake in the oven for 40 to 45 minutes or until set. Take out of the oven afterwards and let completely cool.

Warm strawberries:
1. In a pot, mix the red wine, strawberry extract, cinnamon stick, and remaining swerve sugar. Bring the mixture to a boil and then simmer until the sugar dissolves with occasional stirring.
2. Mix in the strawberries and cook for 10 minutes. Stir in the xanthan gum and cook for 1 minute or until the mixture thickens. Turn the heat off and let slightly cool.
3. Spoon the strawberries with salt on the vanilla pudding and enjoy!

TIPS:
Storage: Chill leftovers in the refrigerator for up to a week.
Reheat: None required.
Serve it with: Swap strawberries for raspberries for a difference in flavor.

NUTRITIONAL FACTS PER SERVING:
Calories: 1059 | Total Fat: 113.38g | Carbs: 7.29g | Fiber: 1.4g | Protein 5.86g

Almond Churro and Chocolate Sauce

Macros: Fat 93% | Protein 3% | Carbs 4%
Prep time: 15 minutes | Cook time: 15 minutes | Serves: 4

Churros are straightforward to assemble but don't ever serve them again without this keto-deserving chocolate sauce. Try it and testify of the goodness.

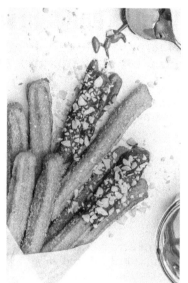

Churros:

1 water
½ cup (113 g) butter
¼ tsp (57 g) salt
½ cup (113 g) swerve sugar
1 ½ cups (340 g) almond flour
4 eggs

Olive oil for frying
A pinch cinnamon powder for garnish
Swerve confectioner's sugar for garnish

Chocolate sauce:

¼ cup coconut cream
¼ cup swerve sugar
1 tsp vanilla extract

3 ½ oz unsweetened dark chocolate, chopped

Churros:

1. In a pot, add the water, butter, salt, and swerve sugar. Bring to a boil and then mix in the almond flour. Reduce the heat to low and cook for 5 to 10 minutes while stirring until the dough is golden brown and comes together.
2. Put the dough into a mixer's bowl, add the eggs and beat until well-incorporated and smooth. Spoon the dough into a star-tripped piping bag.
3. Heat some olive oil in a frying pan over medium heat to deep-fry the churros. Once hot, pipe strips of the dough into the oil and fry on both sides until golden brown. Remove the churros onto a paper towel-lined plate to drain grease. Garnish with some cinnamon powder and swerve confectioner's sugar.

Chocolate sauce:

1. Heat the coconut cream, swerve sugar, and vanilla in a pot over medium heat for 3 to 5 minutes. Turn the heat off and stir in the chocolate until melted and well-combined with the cream mixture.
2. Serve the churros with the chocolate sauce.

TIPS:
Storage: Chill churros and chocolate sauce in the fridge for up to a week.
Reheat: None required.
Serve it with: Swap the chocolate sauce for a sweet cheese sauce for options.

NUTRITIONAL FACTS PER SERVING:
Calories: 1256 | Total Fat: 132.42g | Carbs: 12.06g | Fiber: 2.7g | Protein 7.85g

Pecan Sheet Cake with Sweet Buttercream

Macros: Fat 95% | Protein 4% | Carbs 1%
Prep time: 20 minutes | Cook time: 22 minutes | Serves: 4

A quick cake assemble with a super-creamy topping for a good splurge.

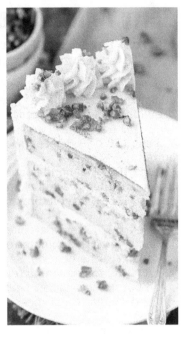

Pecan sheet cake:
2 cups (250 g) almond flour
1 tsp baking powder
¼ tsp salt
2 ½ tbsp unsalted butter, room temperature
1 cup (100 g) erythritol
5 eggs
2 tsp vanilla extract
½ cup (110 g) buttermilk
½ cup (50 g) pecans, chopped

Sweet buttercream:
½ cup (200 g) sugar-free maple syrup
3 egg yolks
A pinch salt
1 tsp vanilla extract
1 tbsp butter, room temperature

Pecan sheet cake:
1. Preheat the oven to 360°F/180°C and line a baking sheet with greaseproof paper. Set aside.
2. Add the almond flour, baking powder, and salt in a bowl and mix well. Set aside.
3. In another bowl, cream the butter and erythritol using beaters until smooth. Add the eggs one at a time while mixing until the batter is smooth, then mix in the vanilla. Pour in the buttermilk and almond flour mixture. Stir well until smooth and fold in the pecans.
4. Pour the mixture into the baking sheet, spread out and evenly layer. Bake in the oven for 20 minutes or until a skewer inserted into the cake comes out with moist crumbs.

Sweet buttercream:
1. Heat the maple syrup in a pot over low heat until reaches a temperature of 250°F/120°C. Take off the heat, cool slightly and whisk in the eggs, and salt until the mixture reaches room temperature.
2. While still whisking, add the vanilla and butter until buttercream forms.
3. Remove the cake from the oven, slightly cool in the sheet and then transfer to a cutting board to completely cool.
4. Spread the buttercream on top, slice and serve.

TIPS:
Storage: Refrigerate leftover cake in the fridge for up to 14 days.
Reheat: None required.
Serve it with: Enjoy the cake with coffee for in-depth flavor.

NUTRITIONAL FACTS PER SERVING:
Calories: 1286 | Total Fat: 137.61g | Carbs: 4.47g | Fiber: 1.2g | Protein 11.16g

Berry Toffee Trifle

Macros: Fat 96% | Protein 1% | Carbs 3%
Prep time: 15 minutes | Cook time: 5 minutes | Serves: 4

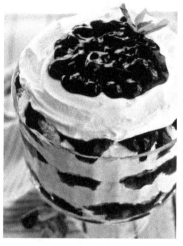

You will do yourself a disfavor by making one serving because it is addictive. Luckily, all the ingredients used are keto-safe, which makes it okay for repeated indulgence.

1/3 cup (70 g) + 1 tbsp unsalted butter
½ cup (100 g) almond flour
2 tbsp chopped toasted almonds
½ cup (125 g) swerve brown sugar

½ cup (125 ml) coconut cream
1 cup (200 g) fresh strawberries, quartered
½ cup (100 g) fresh blueberries
1 ½ c (240 g) heavy cream

1. Melt the butter in a skillet over medium heat and stir-fry the almond flour for 1 to 2 minutes or until toasted. Mix in the toasted almonds and turn the heat off. Set aside to cool.
2. Add the remaining butter, swerve brown sugar, and coconut cream to a pot. Heat over low heat while occasionally stirring until the butter and swerve sugar melts and turns a light amber color. Set aside to cool.
3. To assemble, grab 4 serving bowls. Divide half of the toasted almond flour mixture at the bottom, share half of the heavy cream on top, and drizzle half of the toffee on top. Add some strawberries and blueberries.
4. Repeat the layer a second time in the same manner and enjoy immediately!

TIPS:
Storage: Refrigerate leftover trifle for up to 4 days.
Reheat: None required.
Serve it with: Top the trifle with low-carb biscuits and enjoy!

NUTRITIONAL FACTS PER SERVING:
Calories: 728 | Total Fat: 79.38g | Carbs: 5.75g | Fiber: 0.8g | Protein 1.73g

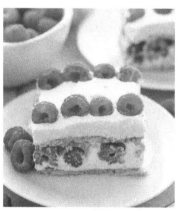

No Bake Lemon Raspberry Pudding

Macros: Fat 93% | Protein 3% | Carbs 4%
Prep time: 10 minutes | Cook time: 5 minutes | Chilling time: 3 hours | Serves: 4

No bake desserts are the best. They come together quickly so that you can enjoy them right after your meal. This pudding is one that you'll love.

2 cups (480 ml) heavy cream
2/3 cup (130 g) swerve sugar
½ lemon, zested and juiced

A pinch salt
Fresh raspberries for serving

TIPS:
Storage: Chill leftovers for up to 3 days.
Reheat: None required.
Serve it with: Top with other berries for a change.

1. In a pot, add the heavy cream, swerve sugar, lemon zest, and salt. Simmer over medium-high heat with frequent whisking for 5 minutes or until the mixture thickens. Turn the heat off and strain the mixture into a measuring cup.
2. Divide the mixture into serving bowls and refrigerate for at least 3 hours.
3. Afterwards, top with the raspberries and enjoy!

NUTRITIONAL FACTS PER SERVING:
Calories: 209 | Total Fat: 22.23g | Carbs: 2.31g | Fiber: 0.1g | Protein 1.27g

Tangy Tiramisu in a Glass

Macros: Fat 92% | Protein 4% | Carbs 4%
Prep time: 20 minutes | Cook time: 0 minutes | Serves: 4

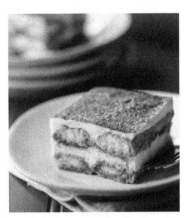

Tiramisu like you never had that features a duo-shade of lemon, cream, and toasted nuts.

2/3 cup (160 g) heavy cream
2/3 cup (160 g) mascarpone cheese
2 tsp vanilla extract
1 tbsp swerve confectioner's sugar

1 tsp fresh lemon zest
1 tsp plain vinegar
4 tbsp unsweetened lemon curd
3 tbsp crushed toasted almonds
1 tbsp toasted cashew nuts

1. In a bowl, add the heavy cream, mascarpone cheese, vanilla extract, swerve confectioner's sugar, lemon zest and vinegar. With beaters, whisk the mixture until frothy.
2. Divide the cream mixture into 4 glasses and top with a tablespoon each of lemon curd. Add the toasted almonds and cashew nuts. Serve immediately!

NUTRITIONAL FACTS PER SERVING:
Calories: 311 | Total Fat: 31.94g | Carbs: 3.11g | Fiber: 0.1g | Protein 3.05g

TIPS:
Storage: Chill leftovers for up to 3 days.
Reheat: None required.
Serve it with: Swirl more whipped cream on the dessert for a creamier effect.

No-Bake Cheesecake Bites

Macros: Fat 89% | Protein 6% | Carbs 5%
Prep time: 20 minutes | Chilling time: 2 hours | Serves: 4

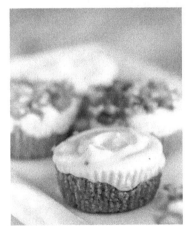

These cheesecake bites take off the burden of baking, almost making you enjoy your dessert in an instant right after combining the ingredients.

1 cup (227 g) walnuts
2 tbsp melted unsalted butter
¼ tsp salt
1 1/3 cups (300 g) cream cheese, room temperature
2/3 cup (150 g) plain yogurt

1 tsp fresh vinegar
1 tsp vanilla extract
½ cup (60 g) swerve confectioner's sugar
½ tbsp (8 g) whipped heavy cream

TIPS:
Storage: Refrigerate leftovers for up to a week.
Reheat: None required.
Serve it with: Top the cake with fresh berries and enjoy better.

1. Add the walnuts, butter, and salt to a blender and process until smooth. Pour the mixture into a springform pan and press the mixture to firm up at the bottom. Set aside.
2. In a clean blender, add the cream cheese, yogurt, vinegar, vanilla extract, swerve confectioner's sugar, and whipped heavy cream. Process until smooth.
3. Pour the mixture over the walnuts and spread out until level on top. Chill the cake in the fridge for at least 2 hours.
4. Afterwards, release the pan, slice the cake into squares and enjoy!

NUTRITIONAL FACTS PER SERVING:
Calories: 524 | Total Fat: 53.35g | Carbs: 6.63g | Fiber: 1.3g | Protein 8.13g

Blackberry Coconut Popsicles

Macros: Fat 92% | Protein 3% | Carbs 5%
Prep time: 5 minutes | Cook time: 10 minutes | Serves: 4

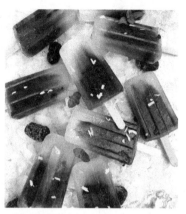

If popsicles were not part of our dessert routine, this cookbook will not be complete. They bring out the childish side of us. It doesn't hurt to be a child now and then.

2 cups (454 g) Greek yogurt
½ cup heavy cream
2/3 cup (159 g) swerve
confectioner's sugar
¼ lemon, juiced
½ cup frozen blackberries

1. In a blender, add the yogurt, heavy cream, swerve confectioner's sugar, vinegar, and blackberries. Process the ingredients until smooth.
2. Pour the mixture into popsicle molds and freeze for at least 6 hours.
3. Enjoy afterwards!

NUTRITIONAL FACTS PER SERVING:
Calories: 265 | Total Fat: 27.8g | Carbs: 3.78g | Fiber: 0.5g | Protein 1.66g

TIPS:
Storage: Keep extras frozen for up to 14 days.
Reheat: None required.
Serve it with: Enjoy as they are!

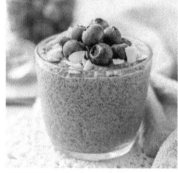

TIPS:
Storage: Chill leftover pudding for up to 3 days.
Reheat: None required.
Serve it with: Top the pudding with some unsweetened coconut flakes for added depth.

Blueberry Chia Pudding

Macros: Fat 95% | Protein 1% | Carbs 4%
Prep time: 10 minutes | Cook time: 0 minutes | Chilling time: overnight | Serves: 4

This pudding is a balance between a breakfast serving and a dessert treat. It is comforting, which either helps you start your day right or calms you for a goodnight sleep.

4 vanilla beans, paste extracted
1 cup (237 ml) almond milk
2 cups (473 ml) coconut milk
4 tbsp sugar-free maple syrup
12 tbsp chia seeds
1 cup (227 g) frozen blueberries, mashed

1. In a bowl, mix the vanilla paste, almond milk, coconut milk, maple syrup, and chia seeds. Divide the mixture into 4 wide glasses and chill overnight.
2. To serve, top with the mashed blueberries and enjoy!

NUTRITIONAL FACTS PER SERVING:
Calories: 724 | Total Fat: 78.85g | Carbs: 7.89g | Fiber: 1g | Protein 2.45g

Coconut Matcha Ice Cream

Macros: Fat 88% | Protein 8% | Carbs 4%
Prep time: 20 minutes | Cooking time: 4 minutes |
Freezing time: 18 hours | Serves: 4

Try this coconut matcha version for alternative flavors.

1 cup (250 ml) coconut cream
½ cup (150 ml) coconut milk
¼ cup xylitol
3 tsp matcha powder

4 egg yolks
2 ½ tbsp sugar-free maple syrup
¼ tsp plain vinegar
Ice cubes

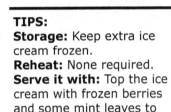

1. Beat half of the coconut cream in a bowl until stiff. Set aside.
2. Add the remaining coconut cream and coconut milk to a pot. Place over medium heat and once simmering, whisk in the xylitol and matcha powder until well-combined. Simmer for 1 more minute and turn the heat off.
3. Pour the egg yolks, maple syrup, and vinegar in a bowl. Place the bowl on top of a pot of boiling water. Whisk for 3 to 4 minutes or until thickened. Make sure not to overheat to prevent the eggs from cooking.
4. After, mix with matcha cream and then, the coconut cream until smooth mixture forms. Freeze the mixture for 15 to 18 hours.
5. Scoop the ice cream into bowls and enjoy!

TIPS:
Storage: Keep extra ice cream frozen.
Reheat: None required.
Serve it with: Top the ice cream with frozen berries and some mint leaves to improve the taste.

NUTRITIONAL FACTS PER SERVING:
Calories: 214 | Total Fat: 21.64g | Carbs: 2.24g | Fiber: 0g | Protein 3.88g

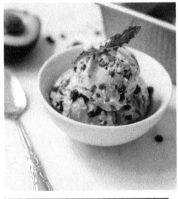

Avo-Blueberry Ice Cream

Macros: Fat 95% | Protein 1% | Carbs 4%
Prep time: 10 minutes | Freezing time: overnight | Serves: 4

An easy way to construct ice cream without bananas or an ice cream machine.

1 cup (237 ml) almond milk
1 cup heavy cream
1 tbsp sugar-free maple syrup

¼ avocado, peeled and pitted
1 cups (227 g) frozen blueberries

1. Mix the almond milk, heavy cream, and maple syrup, and fill one or two ice cube trays with the mixture. Freeze overnight.
2. The next day, empty the frozen coconut milk, avocado, and blueberries into a blender. Process at high speed until creamy.
3. Scoop the mixture into bowls and enjoy!

TIPS:
Storage: Keep extra ice cream frozen.
Reheat: None required.
Serve it with: Garnish the ice cream with mint leaves to introduce hints of peppermint into each bite.

NUTRITIONAL FACTS PER SERVING:
Calories: 625 | Total Fat: 67.69g | Carbs: 6.63g | Fiber: 1.9g | Protein 1.03g

Almond Turmeric Drink

Macros: Fat 99% | Protein 0% | Carbs 1%
Prep time: 5 minutes | Cook time: 5 minutes | Serves: 4

An enticing glass that calls out for a long slip. The color and flavor of this drink sends cheerful notes whenever consumed.

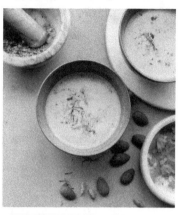

1 cup (240 ml) water
1 tsp turmeric
¼ tsp nutmeg powder
¼ tsp ginger powder

2 cups (933 ml) almond milk
2 cups (480 ml) heavy cream
4 tbsp sugar-free maple syrup
1 tsp cinnamon powder

1. Mix the water and turmeric in a pot and heat over medium heat. Once boiling, stir in the nutmeg powder and ginger powder. Continue boiling until the mixture reduces to a paste.
2. Whisk in the almond milk, heavy cream, maple syrup, and cinnamon powder. Cook for 2 minutes and turn the heat off.
3. Pour the drink into mugs, sift some cinnamon powder on top and enjoy.

NUTRITIONAL FACTS PER SERVING:
Calories: 1175 | Total Fat: 131.29g | Carbs: 2.8g | Fiber: 0.5g | Protein 1.34g

TIPS:
Storage: Refrigerate leftover drink
Reheat: Enjoy chilled or warm in the microwave.
Serve it with: Add the drink to a pre-brunch routine or enjoy as a working or relaxation snack.

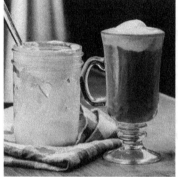

Irish No-Alcohol Coffee

Macros: Fat 93% | Protein 3% | Carbs 4%
Prep time: 10 minutes | Cook time: 5 minutes | Serves: 4

Irish coffee is a classic at many cafes. However, for the sake of the keto diet and not losing out on the good treat, this no alcohol version will satisfy just as much.

6 oz (170 g) ground coffee
5 ½ cups (1301 ml) water
2 tbsp sugar-free maple syrup

1 tsp pure vanilla extract
4 tbsp heavy cream
Ice cubes for serving

1. Brew the coffee with the water in a coffee maker.
2. Divide the drink between four glasses and stir in maple syrup, vanilla extract, and heavy cream.
3. Add some ice cubes to the glass and enjoy chilled.

NUTRITIONAL FACTS PER SERVING:
Calories: 55 | Total Fat: 5.56g | Carbs: 0.55g | Fiber: 0 g | Protein 0.36g

TIPS:
Storage: Chill leftover drink in a jar or bottle for up to a week.
Reheat: None required.
Serve it with: Add coffee drink to your breakfast serving for a more satisfying fill.

Chocolate Matcha Latte

Macros: Fat 94% | Protein 3% | Carbs 3%
Prep time: 10 minutes | Cook time: 1 minute | Serves: 4

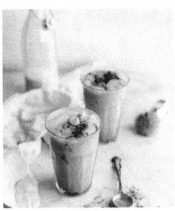

Asian vibes burst out of these cups, screaming a healthy presence. Coconut milk and matcha powder are a happy pair; hence, you will love every sip of this drink.

3 ¼ cups (769 ml) unsweetened coconut milk
¾ cup (177 ml) water

½ tsp vanilla extract
1 tsp matcha powder
4 tbsp unsweetened cocoa powder

1. In a pot, mix the coconut milk, water, and vanilla extract. Warm over low heat for 1 minute and mix well.
2. Turn the heat off and stir in matcha powder and cocoa powder. Mix well.
3. Pour the drink into cups and enjoy!

NUTRITIONAL FACTS PER SERVING:
Calories: 340 | Total Fat: 36.08g | Carbs: 3.26g | Fiber: 0.1g | Protein 2.06g

TIPS:
Storage: Chill excess drink in a jar for up to a week.
Reheat: None required.
Serve it with: Pair the drink with some seeds crackers for better snacking.

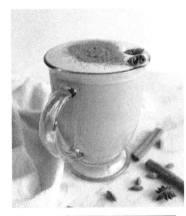

Coconut Vanilla Chai

Macros: Fat 91% | Protein 4% | Carbs 6%
Prep time: 10 minutes | Cook time: 4 minutes | Serves: 4

If you aren't sure of what to make with your black tea bags, try this tea blend. It is creamy, aromatic, and passes all the marks for the keto diet.

1 cup (237 ml) water
4 black tea bags
20 cardamom pods
4 cinnamon sticks
4 star anise

8 cloves
½ tsp ginger paste
3 cups (710 ml) unsweetened coconut milk
2 tbsp sugar-free maple syrup

TIPS:
Storage: Chill leftover tea in a jar for up to 5 days.
Reheat: None required.
Serve it with: Pair the drink with some seeds crackers for better snacking.

1. Add the water to a pot and bring to a boil. Turn the heat off and stir in the tea bags, cardamom pods, cinnamon sticks, star anise, cloves, and ginger. Let steep for 2 to 3 minutes and strain the drink.
2. Stir the coconut milk and maple syrup into the liquid and divide the drink into 4 cups. Enjoy immediately!

NUTRITIONAL FACTS PER SERVING:
Calories: 445 | Total Fat: 48.21g | Carbs: 6.4g | Fiber: 0g | Protein 4.57g

Blueberry Pistachio Smoothie

Macros: Fat 93% | Protein 3% | Carbs 4%
Prep time: 10 minutes | Cook time: 0 minutes | Serves: 4

Berries may not be heavily encouraged for dieting at this age. However, when you want to splurge on a bit, this pistachio-supporting smoothie is one to go down deliciously. The recipes below also share other unique ways for using berries when needed. Check them out!

¼ cup (56.5g) frozen blueberries   4 cups heavy cream
1 tsp pistachios

1. In a blender, add the blueberries, pistachios, and heavy cream. Process until smooth.
2. Divide the smoothie between 4 glasses and enjoy!

NUTRITIONAL FACTS PER SERVING:
Calories: 423 | Total Fat: 44.76g | Carbs: 4.71g | Fiber: 0.3g | Protein 2.63g

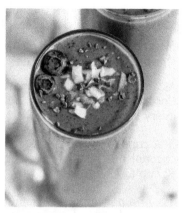

TIPS:
Storage: Preferably, enjoy the smoothie freshly blended. Chill any extra and add it to a new blend.
Reheat: None required.
Serve it with: Enjoy as a snack or as a quick pre-breakfast drink.

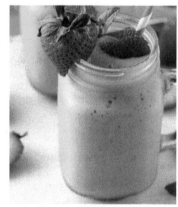

Red Creamy Smoothie

Macros: Fat 93% | Protein 3% | Carbs 4%
Prep time: 10 minutes | Cook time: 0 minutes | Serves: 4

This smoothie reminds us of the many red riding hood cocktails we enjoyed outdoors when not on the keto diet. To bring in a bit of that vibe into your home, make this red creamy blend of a smoothie.

¼ cup (56.5g) frozen raspberries   3 ½ cups (473 ml) heavy cream
and strawberries   3 tbsp unsweetened coconut milk
½ lemon, juiced   Mint leaves to garnish

1. Combine all the ingredients in a blender and process until smooth.
2. Divide the smoothie into 4 serving glasses, garnish with the mint leaves and enjoy!

NUTRITIONAL FACTS PER SERVING:
Calories: 389 | Total Fat: 41.26g | Carbs: 4.51g | Fiber: 0.3g | Protein 2.44g

TIPS:
Storage: Preferably, enjoy the smoothie freshly blended. Chill any extra and add it to a new blend.
Reheat: None required.
Serve it with: Enjoy as a snack or as a quick pre-breakfast drink.

Cinnamon Peanut Butter Smoothie

Macros: Fat 92% | Protein 3% | Carbs 5%
Prep time: 10 minutes | Cook time: 0 minutes | Serves: 4

Peanut butter with heavy cream are loaded with amazing fatty elements. When not spreading peanut butter on your low-carb toasts, you can make a creamy smoothie out of it. Enjoy the splurge!

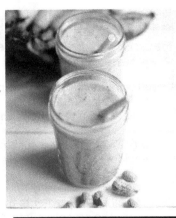

¼ avocado
3 ¼ cup heavy cream
1 tbsp pure peanut butter
1 lemon, juiced

1 tsp vanilla extract
¼ cup (59 ml) almond milk
Cinnamon powder to garnish

1. In a blender, add the avocado, heavy cream, peanut butter, vinegar, vanilla, and almond milk. Process until smooth.
2. Pour the drink into 4 serving glasses, garnish with the cinnamon powder and enjoy!

NUTRITIONAL FACTS PER SERVING:
Calories: 435 | Total Fat: 45.18g | Carbs: 5.61g | Fiber: 0.9g | Protein 3.59g

TIPS:
Storage: For a better taste, have the smoothie freshly blended. Chill any extra and add it to a new blend.
Reheat: None required.
Serve it with: Enjoy as a snack or as a quick pre-breakfast drink.

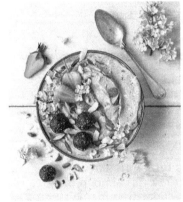

Dreamy Chocolate Strawberry Smoothie

Macros: Fat 92% | Protein 3% | Carbs 5%
Prep time: 10 minutes | Cook time: 0 minutes | Serves: 4

Luckily, chocolate is welcomed on the keto diet and very much allowed after over fifty years of age. Therefore, to have chocolate in a healthy way, this creamy chocolate smoothie serves right. It features some strawberries, which you can exclude if you are not up for berries.

¼ cup (57 g) frozen strawberries
1 tbsp pecans
1 tsp vanilla extract
4 tbsp unsweetened cocoa powder
1 tsp cinnamon powder

1 cup (355 ml) unsweetened coconut milk
3 cups (237 ml) heavy cream
Ice cubes

1. Add all the ingredients to a blender and process until smooth.
2. Pour the smoothie into 4 glasses and enjoy immediately.

NUTRITIONAL FACTS PER SERVING:
Calories: 446 | Total Fat: 46.85g | Carbs: 6.73g | Fiber: 1.2g | Protein 3.48g

TIPS:
Storage: It is better to enjoy the smoothie freshly blended for the best taste. Chill any extra and add it to a new blend.
Reheat: None required.
Serve it with: Enjoy as a snack or as a quick pre-breakfast drink.

Avo-Cucumber Smoothie

Macros: Fat 94% | Protein 2% | Carbs 4%
Prep time: 10 minutes | Cook time: 0 minutes | Serves: 4

Cucumbers have an unfair reputation as a salad ingredient only. You can make drinks out of them and enjoy the therapeutic aroma that they offer. Blending a few chops with avocado makes for an excellent drink.

1 cup (227 g) chopped cucumbers
¼ avocados, pitted and peeled
1 ½ cup (237 ml) almond milk
½ cup unsweetened coconut milk
2 cups (473 ml) Greek yogurt
1 lime, juiced

1. Add all the ingredients to a blender and process until smooth.
2. Share the smoothie into 4 serving glasses and enjoy immediately!

NUTRITIONAL FACTS PER SERVING:
Calories: 879 | Total Fat: 93.66g | Carbs: 9.14g | Fiber: 1.1g | Protein 5.29g

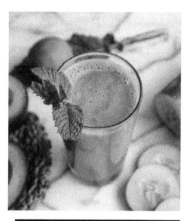

TIPS:
Storage: It is better to enjoy the smoothie freshly blended for the best taste. Chill any extra and add it to a new blend.
Reheat: None required.
Serve it with: Enjoy as a snack or as a quick pre-breakfast drink.

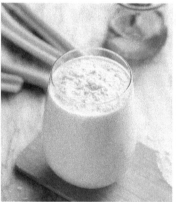

Coconut Celery Smoothie

Macros: Fat 97% | Protein 1% | Carbs 2%
Prep time: 10 minutes | Cook time: 0 minutes | Serves: 4

The smell of celery may be overpowering, however, it offers tremendous health benefits. It is an excellent option for detox when trying weight loss. Hence, this smoothie that includes coconut milk and cream serves as the right pair for celery to reduce its intense flavor. This way, you can reap all the benefits of celery accurately.

1 celery stick, roughly chopped
1 cup (474 ml) unsweetened coconut milk
2 cups (237 ml) heavy cream
1 cup (237 ml) almond milk
2 tbsp sugar-free maple syrup

1. Add all the ingredients to a blender and process until smooth.
2. Pour the smoothie into 4 serving glasses and enjoy immediately.

NUTRITIONAL FACTS PER SERVING:
Calories: 804 | Total Fat: 88.79g | Carbs: 4.01g | Fiber: 0.4g | Protein 2.55g

TIPS:
Storage: For a fresh taste, enjoy the smoothie the same moment. Otherwise, chill any extras and use it to reconstruct a new smoothie.
Reheat: None required.
Serve it with: Enjoy as a snack or as a quick pre-breakfast drink.

Black Sesame Smoothie

Macros: Fat 96% | Protein 1% | Carbs 3%
Prep time: 10 minutes | Cook time: 0 minutes | Serves: 4

Black sesame seeds uniquely decorate sushi pieces and may not be incorporated in many American diets. This drink is one smart way to use black sesame seeds while filling up on all its good nutrients.

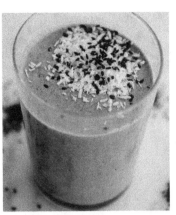

1 ½ tbsp black sesame seeds
1 avocado
2 cups almond milk
1 ½ cups macadamia nut milk

¼ cup unsweetened grated coconut
2 tbsp sugar-free maple syrup
A pinch of salt

1. Ground the sesame seeds in spice blender until smooth.
2. Add the sesame powder to a bigger blender and pour in the remaining ingredients. Process until smooth.
3. Divide the smoothie into 4 serving cups and enjoy!

NUTRITIONAL FACTS PER SERVING:
Calories: 1305 | Total Fat: 143.6g | Carbs: 9.55g | Fiber: 6.7g | Protein 4.32g

TIPS:
Storage: Enjoy the smoothie fresh for better tastes. Otherwise, refrigerate for up to a week and use it to reconstruct another smoothie.
Reheat: None required.
Serve it with: Have the smoothie as a snack or a pre-breakfast treat.

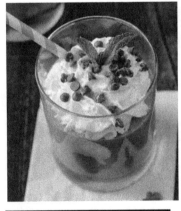

Hemp Shamrock Shake

Macros: Fat 97% | Protein 1% | Carbs 2%
Prep time: 10 minutes | Cook time: 0 minutes | Serves: 4

Grab some mint leaves, flavoring, avocado, and heavy cream, and make a shamrock shake that wins! It is an excellent pre-breakfast serve as well as a quick lunch fill-up.

2 cups (474 ml) unsweetened almond milk
1 ½ cups (357 ml) heavy cream
1 avocado, pitted and peeled
¼ tsp mint extract

4 fresh mint leaves
2 tbsp hulled hemp seeds
3 tbsp erythritol
A pinch of sea salt
1 cup (227 g) ice cubes

TIPS:
Storage: Enjoy the smoothie fresh for a better taste. You may refrigerate extras for up to a week and use it to reconstruct another smoothie.
Reheat: None required.
Serve it with: Have the smoothie as a snack or a pre-breakfast treat.

1. Add all the ingredients to a blender and process until smooth.
2. Divide the drink into 4 serving glasses and enjoy!

NUTRITIONAL FACTS PER SERVING:
Calories: 1226 | Total Fat: 135.27g | Carbs: 6.45g | Fiber: 3.7g | Protein 2.84g

White Russian

Macros: Fat 93% | Protein 4% | Carbs 3%
Prep time: 10 minutes | Cook time: 0 minutes | Serves: 2

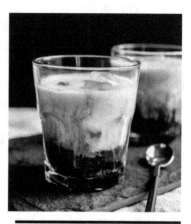

Vodka is permitted on the keto diet but does not add any nutritional benefits to your body. However, if you would like to introduce some alcohol into your routine, this drink incorporates vodka with many nutritional benefits.

2 cups brewed coffee, chilled
2 tbsp vodka
2 tbsp sugar-free maple syrup

3 tbsp heavy cream
Ice cubes for serving

1. In a jar, mix the coffee, vodka, and maple syrup.
2. Divide the ice cubes into 4 serving cups and pour on the coffee mixture. Divide the heavy cream into the drink and serve immediately!

NUTRITIONAL FACTS PER SERVING:
Calories: 40 | Total Fat: 4.19g | Carbs: 0.31g | Fiber: 0g | Protein 0.37g

TIPS:
Storage: Chill extra drink in the refrigerator for up to 5 days.
Reheat: None required.
Serve it with: Compliment lunch or dinner dishes with this drink.

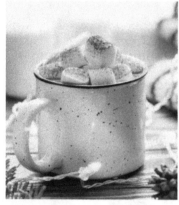

American Hot Chocolate

Macros: Fat 93% | Protein 3% | Carbs 4%
Prep time: 10 minutes | Cook time: 4 minutes | Serves: 2

Enjoy this keto version of hot chocolate and reap the healthy fatty benefits at the same time.

1 ½ cups (355 ml) hot water
1 cup (118 ml) heavy cream + extra for topping
4 pieces unsweetened 100% chocolate, finely chopped

2 heaped tbsp unsweetened cocoa powder
½ tsp cinnamon powder
2 scoops keto collagen
Swerve sugar to taste

1. Add the hot water and heavy cream to a pot and simmer for 1 to 2 minutes. Turn the heat off.
2. Stir in the chocolate and cocoa powder until melted. Add the cinnamon powder, keto collagen and swerve sugar. Mix well.
3. Divide the mixture into 4 serving cups, top with some heavy cream and enjoy!

NUTRITIONAL FACTS PER SERVING:
Calories: 107 | Total Fat: 11.28g | Carbs: 1.62g | Fiber: 0.5g | Protein 0.88g

TIPS:
Storage: Chill extra hot chocolate in the fridge for up to a day.
Reheat: Warm in the microwave.
Serve it with: Add hot chocolate to your breakfast routine and enjoy!

Appendix1: Measurement Conversion Chart

VOLUME EQUIVALENTS(DRY)

US STANDARD	METRIC (APPROXIMATE)
1/8 teaspoon	0.5 mL
1/4 teaspoon	1 mL
1/2 teaspoon	2 mL
3/4 teaspoon	4 mL
1 teaspoon	5 mL
1 tablespoon	15 mL
1/4 cup	59 mL
1/2 cup	118 mL
3/4 cup	177 mL
1 cup	235 mL
2 cups	475 mL
3 cups	700 mL
4 cups	1 L

WEIGHT EQUIVALENTS

US STANDARD	METRIC (APPROXIMATE)
1 ounce	28 g
2 ounces	57 g
5 ounces	142 g
10 ounces	284 g
15 ounces	425 g
16 ounces (1 pound)	455 g
1.5 pounds	680 g
2 pounds	907 g

VOLUME EQUIVALENTS(LIQUID)

US STANDARD	US STANDARD (OUNCES)	METRIC (APPROXIMATE)
2 tablespoons	1 fl.oz.	30 mL
1/4 cup	2 fl.oz.	60 mL
1/2 cup	4 fl.oz.	120 mL
1 cup	8 fl.oz.	240 mL
1 1/2 cup	12 fl.oz.	355 mL
2 cups or 1 pint	16 fl.oz.	475 mL
4 cups or 1 quart	32 fl.oz.	1 L
1 gallon	128 fl.oz.	4 L

TEMPERATURES EQUIVALENTS

FAHRENHEIT(F)	CELSIUS(C) (APPROXIMATE)
225 °F	107 °C
250 °F	120 °C
275 °F	135 °C
300 °F	150 °C
325 °F	160 °C
350 °F	180 °C
375 °F	190 °C
400 °F	205 °C
425 °F	220 °C
450 °F	235 °C
475 °F	245 °C
500 °F	260 °C

References

AsiaOne. (n.d.). Is it normal to menstruate when I'm over 50-years-old? https://www.asiaone.com/health/it-normal-menstruate-when-im-over-50yearsold

Branco, A.F., Ferreira, A., Simoes, R.F., Magalhaes-Novais, S., Zehowski, C., Cope, E., Silva, A.M., Pareira, D., Sardao, V.A. & Cunha-Oliveira, T. (2016). Ketogenic diets: From cancer to mitochondrial diseases and beyond. PubMed. https://pubmed.ncbi.nlm.nih.gov/26782788/

Bryce. E. (2019). How many calories can the brain burn by thinking? LiveScience. https://www.livescience.com/burn-calories-brain.html

Calculator.net. (n.d.). Calorie Calculator. https://www.calculator.net/calorie-calculator.html

Campos, M. (2017). Ketogenic diet: Is the ultimate low-carb diet good for you? Harvard health publishing. https://www.health.harvard.edu/blog/ketogenic-diet-is-the-ultimate-low-carb-diet-good-for-you-2017072712089

Centres for Disease Control and Prevention. (n.d.). PCOS (Polycystic ovarian syndrome) and diabetes. https://www.cdc.gov/diabetes/basics/pcos.html

Cohen, C.W., Fontaine, K.R., Arend, R.C., Alvarez, R.D., Leath III, C.A., Hun, W.K., Bevis, K.S., Kim, K.H., Straughn, J.M. & Gower, B.A. (2018). A ketogenic diet reduces central obesity and serum insulin in women with ovarian or endometrial cancer. The Journal of Nutrition, 148(8), 1253-1260. https://doi.org/10.1093/jn/nxy119

Cox, N., Gibas, S., Salisbury, M., Gomer, J. & Gibas, K. (2019). Ketogenic diets potentially reverse type 2 diabetes and ameliorate clinical depression: A case study. Diabetes Metabolic Syndrome, 13(2), 1475-1479. http://doi.org/10.1016/j.dsx.2019.01.055

Davis, S.R., Castelo-Branco, C., Chedraui, P., Lumsden, M., Nappy, R.E., Shan, D. & Villaseca, P. (2012). Understanding weight gain at menopause. National Library of Medicine. https://pubmed.ncbi.nlm.nih.gov/22978257/

Dyson, P. (2015). Low Carbohydrate Diets and Type 2 Diabetes: What is the Latest Evidence? U.S. National Library of Medicine National Institute of Health. https://www.ncbi.nlm.nih.gov/pmc/articles/PMC4674467/

Goday, A., Bellido, D., Sajoux, I., Crujeiras, A.B., Burqeura, B., Garcia-Luna, P.P., Oleaga, A., Moreno, B. & Casaneuva, F.F. (2016). Short-term safety, tolerability and efficacy of a very low-calorie-ketogenic diet interventional weight loss program versus hypocaloric diet in patients with type 2 diabetes mellitus. Nutritional Diabetes, 6(9), 230. https://www.ncbi.nlm.nih.gov/pmc/articles/PMC5048014/

Jackson, T. (2017). High-Fat vs High-Carbohydrate Diet and Cardiovascular Disease: Which diet offers more heart protection?Natural Medicine Journal, 9(11). https://www.naturalmedicinejournal.com/journal/2017-11/high-fat-vs-high-carbohydrate-diet-and-cardiovascular-disease

Manikam, N., Pantoro, N., Komala, K. & Sari, A. (2018). Comparing the efficacy of ketogenic diet with low-fat diet for weight loss in obesity Patients: Evidence-based case report. Research Gate. https://www.researchgate.net/publication/327189134_Comparing_the_Efficacy_of_Ketogenic_Diet_with_Low-Fat_Diet_for_Weight_Loss_in_Obesity_Patients_Evidenc-Based_Case_Report

Massod, W., Annamaraju, P. & Uppulari, K.R. (2020). Ketogenic diet. NCBI. https://www.ncbi.nlm.nih.gov/books/NBK499830/

McGrice, M & Porter, J. (2017). The effect of low carbohydrate diets on fertility hormones and outcomes in overweight and obese women: A systematic review. Nutrients, 9(3), 204. https://doi.org.10.3390/nu9030204

Redman, L.M., Smith, S.R., Burton, J.H.Martin, C.K, Il'yasova, D. & Ravussin, E. (2018). Metabolic slowing and reduced oxidative damage with sustained caloric restriction supports the rate of living and oxidative damage theories of aging. Cell Metab, 27(4), 805-815. https://doi.org/10.1016/j.cmet.2018.02.019

Zampelas, Z. & Magriplis, E. (2019) New Insights into Cholesterol Functions: A Friend or an Enemy? National Library of Medicine National Institute of Health. https://www.ncbi.nlm.nih.gov/pmc/articles/PMC6682969/

CPSIA information can be obtained
at www.ICGtesting.com
Printed in the USA
LVHW060836121020
668068LV00056B/50